T0328036

Plants for the People

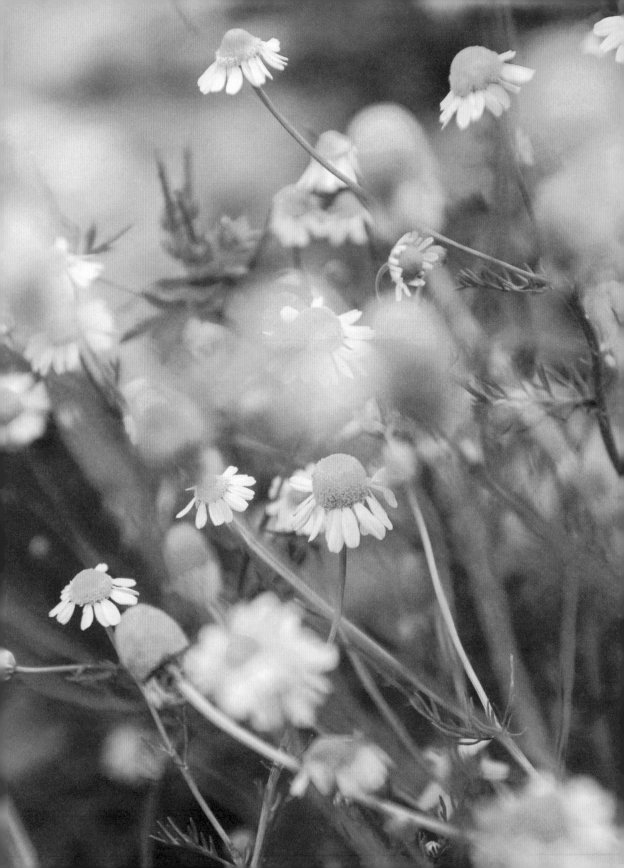

Plants
for
the
People

A modern guide
to plant medicine

Erin Lovell Verinder

B HERB MED, ADV DIP NUT MED, DIP ENERGY HEALING

PART 3

MATERIA MEDICA 111

Contents

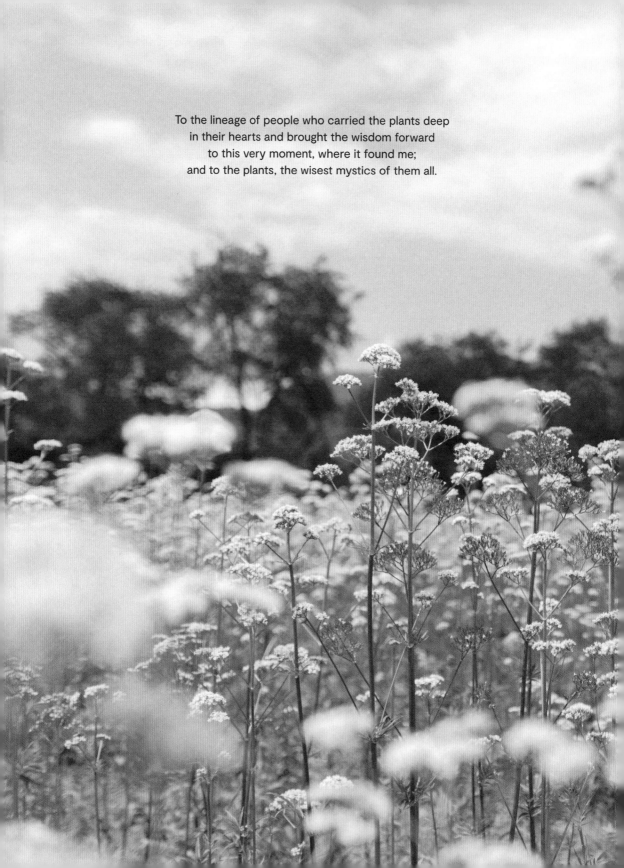

To the lineage of people who carried the plants deep
in their hearts and brought the wisdom forward
to this very moment, where it found me;
and to the plants, the wisest mystics of them all.

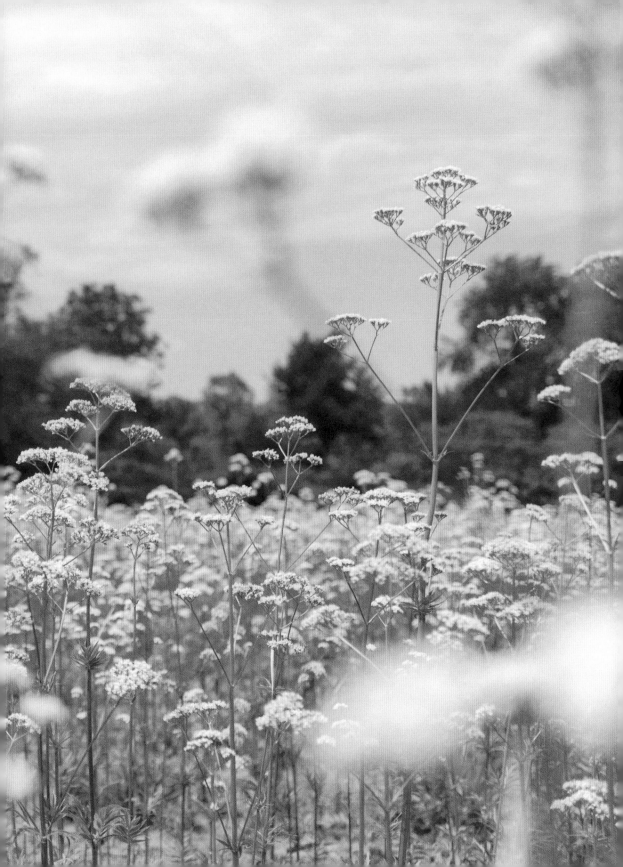

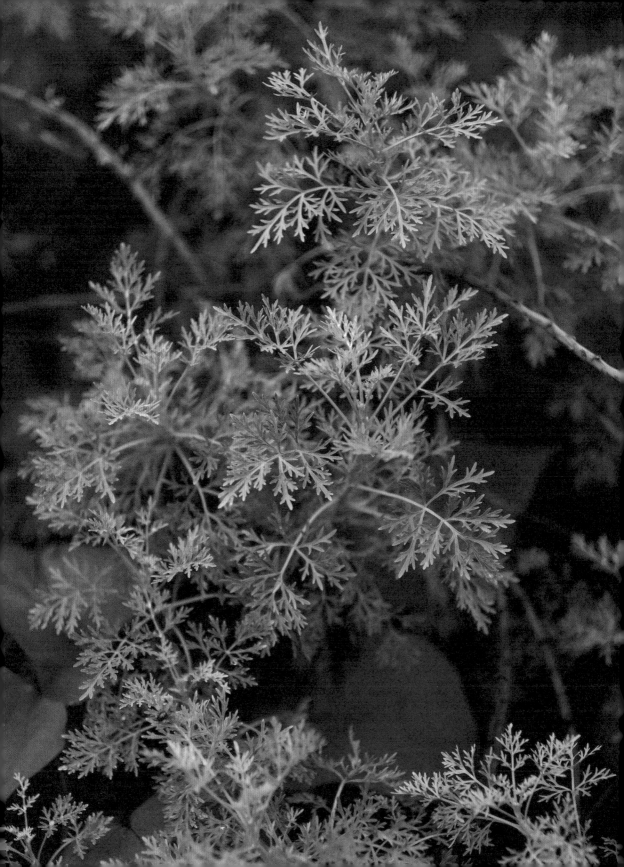

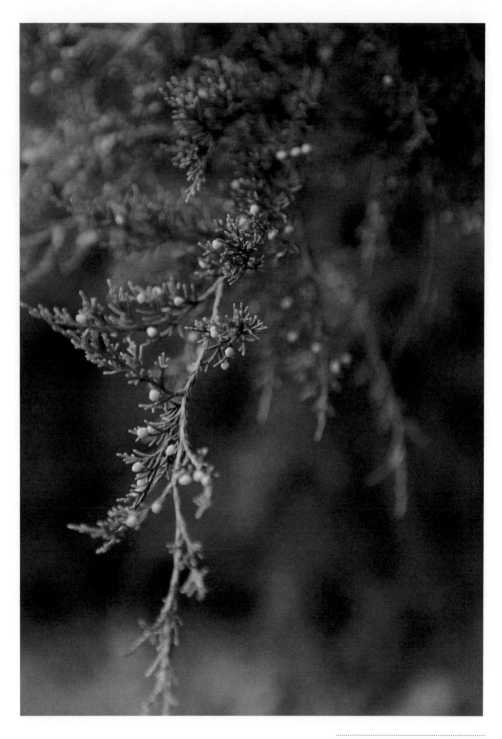

ABOVE: Juniper berries ripening

LEFT: Wormwood, full of might

INTRODUCTION

If you were lucky enough to be raised with plant whisperers and folk remedies, frolicking in the meadows and under the oak trees, I am sincerely happy for you. Albeit a little envious.

Most of us in this modern day, including myself, were raised more around electronics and concrete jungles. Your experience of the natural world may have been fleeting and tame, not wild and connected. Perhaps there was little knowledge of or encouragement to commune with nature.

I grew up in a coiffed suburban area, where gardens were cultivated and tended to, lawns mowed and edged. Where 'weeds' were treated with annoyance and there was not an iota of herbicide-free spray in sight. It was the 80s; there was nothing medicinal about a 'weed' in the suburbs!

Yet I had a keen feel for nature. I never wanted to wear shoes as a child. I trusted that I would be just fine navigating the world barefoot. I didn't mind the hazards of stinging insects, spiky grasses, sun-punched asphalt roads – gratefully exhaling with relief as I plunged my bare feet into a patch of sunny yellow dandelion flowers.

This is where I first encountered plant medicine.

I met the milky stalks of dandelion (*Taraxacum officinale*) on the front lawn, the hairy stems and erect flower heads of ribwort plantain (*Plantago lanceolata*) in the field up the road, the sweet nectar of Japanese honeysuckle (*Lonicera japonica*) in my best friend's garden, the tangled vines and brilliant flowers of jasmine (*Jasminum polyanthum*) growing over our fence, and the sticky marvel of cleavers (*Galium aparine*) catching my uniform on the school oval.

Despite the efforts of many avid gardeners and even governments, these 'weeds' and plants grow. Everywhere.

I will speculate as far as to say that most of you holding this book heard whispers of the healing abilities of plants in your upbringing. Perhaps Grandma used to prepare sage-leaf gargles for a sore throat, fresh aloe vera was applied to a knee scrape, or when a tummy ache set in, ginger tea was made and served. These traditions, likely passed down through many generations, always seem to hold a magical quality, a soothing, familiar essence. This is the spirit of traditional plant medicine. Sadly, much has been forgotten in our everyday approach to plants, health and healing.

In our modern age, we have perhaps been led to overlook the riches of nature. Our innate connection to the land we live on is often devastatingly broken. We may not quite feel native to any place, let alone in harmony with the heartbeat of the plant kingdom around us.

There is a call. The collective call is to return to the simple way. To know your body. To thrive rather than succumb to the epidemic of strung-out nervous systems, anxiety, depression and depleted reserves causing chronic illness, the rise of autoimmune conditions, and intolerance of the fast-paced urban environments many of us live in. For most of us, the 'normal' modern day consists of rush, compression, stimulation, multitasking, more rushing, rinse and repeat. Stress is a natural by-product of keeping up such a frenetic pace, and unfortunately it causes many expressions of ill health. It is therefore more important than ever to find ways to activate self-care, vitality and wellness.

What if we were to know the medicines that aid and support our bodies? The antidote to the body 'on edge', the sleepless nights, the reactive digestive system. Plant medicine attunes to our needs the way only nature can, offering essential healing elements for body, mind and soul. This is the return to simplicity, the return to nature.

With the ever-growing global wellness movement, we are seeking to improve ourselves, our environments and our quality of life. To understand where and why our health goes awry, we are turning to ancient knowledge and practices, with thirsty minds and parched bodies. We are turning to the plants for answers.

Science is continually affirming us naturalists. We are an educated society, so naturally research gives many faith. Countless studies are confirming the medicinal powers of plants and the effect nature has on our health. Research shows that having a green home or workplace, or spending time in nature, physiologically reduces stress and enhances positive attitudes. Many of us do not need research to tell us we feel alive and that every cell in our body sings when we go out into the wild green expanse. But some do need this confirmation. Regardless of how down to earth you may be, the good news is that collectively we are realigning to nature's way.

Plant medicine invites you to return to the roots, to aid recalibration of your body and being. To shift from feeling disempowered in your own experience of health, and ultimately, to assist with the reclamation of your personal version of wellness. What we often overlook is that we are all so individual. There is no one type of healthy, or balanced, or well. And regardless of all the experts out there on health and wellness, you are your best compass. We are all deeply individualistic, with our stories of how we came to be – multifaceted, needing different elements and conditions to thrive. As a herbalist, I am well versed in plant medicine, and as a practitioner I am well versed in humanity. Finding the attuned plant remedies for a client is a beautiful process, and the perfection of a match is the most rewarding outcome. Alchemy happens; health is transformed from this space. People get better.

Harnessing the powers of plants for medicine is our oldest known system of healing. Hippocrates, the ancient Greek physician and father of medicine, had it right when he said: 'Nature itself is the best physician.' Gardens of medicinal plants have been kept for eons, and wild plants have been foraged for the health of communities for as long as we have been here, in one way or another. The bottom line is that our origin story of healing begins with the plants.

I began my earthy education learning how to grow things from my uncle, a jolly Englishman who had served in the navy but found his best medicine was with the basil and the bees. My uncle was once a fruiterer. He had a kinship with his garden and the produce that came from it. Not only did I learn how important the plants were to him, I witnessed the joy that flowed from him when he was in communion with them. I observed the importance of cultivating the soil, watering the crop and harvesting in a timely manner. How sometimes the carrots would be gnarled and intertwined, but they still tasted like paradise. Gardening seemed like the ultimate metaphor for life's lessons. Those muddy sessions taught me that the earth was wise, and worked in mysterious ways, and that with a little gentle support you could feel a part of it all. This caught my attention, and I wondered what other pearls the dirt held.

I always trusted that the answers to our ill health would be rooted in the soils, and I recall feeling misplaced learning about the incredible green world of herbs within four walls, sitting behind a desk, looking at a whiteboard. I yearned for the plants to come to life from my textbook pages. I desired to understand their personalities, their abilities and uniqueness, and saw that my clinical training was missing something. It missed the softness and connected spirit. And so I began to bridge the gaps, weaving the spirit with the science, the folk traditions with the knowing.

I have spent years walking this plant path. In addition to studying extensively in the traditional sense, I have studied under incredible herbalists, naturopaths and healers. I have been privileged to work in clinical practice, witnessing health transformations daily, and to teach the powers of plants to rooms full of eager eyes and ears. I have spent time growing plants, out wildcrafting in the woods, mastering infusion combinations and creating the perfect creams.

I continue to work at the intersection of clinical naturopathic medicine, grassroots plant medicine and intuitive healing. In essence, I empower my clients to understand that physical symptoms are the gateway, and that we have an innate ability to shift our health stories with the assistance of nature and all her breathtaking powers.

We exist in a time plagued by separation from nature, riddled with suppressing the wildness within ourselves. A wonderful opportunity exists for us to craft a relationship with the wild through the medicinal plant path, to bring it into our hearts, our homes. We all come from the great green spaces, and you know full well you were not born to be tame.

An elder once told me her mentor took her deep into the forest and said to her, 'Lie belly-down on the ground with your face in the earth, and do not get up until the dirt smells sweet.'

You cannot learn this in a classroom – you have to step into your wild.

Understanding that the earth holds the remedies is a great perspective shift. Not only is attuning to the healing properties of plants a gift to yourself, it also sows the seeds for the tradition of plant medicine to live on. And most importantly, it creates a relationship with the greatest mother of them all, the earth.

Plant medicine is your birthright, and the opportunity it offers to be in a relationship with the natural world is a mighty potent solution to the times we exist in. So many plant medicines are in vogue these days – the new super-herb, superfood, super tonic. In truth, many of the most potent remedies are common – not so flashy and new, but age-old.

In these pages, I hope to lay foundations for you to understand that we have the greatest plant allies to support us, often growing right nearby. I hope to deliver you crystal-clear guidance along with accessible insights, so that this becomes a book you treasure. You have been called to the plant path. It is the most extraordinary road to travel.

This book is not intended to replace individualised professional advice on healthcare and wellbeing. Its aim is to offer a helpful guide to plant medicine, and as such it is not meant to be utilised to diagnose, or treat. It is recommended that you consult your naturopathic practitioner or herbalist when seeking natural healthcare support: health runs deep, and there is no such thing as a one-size-fits-all approach.

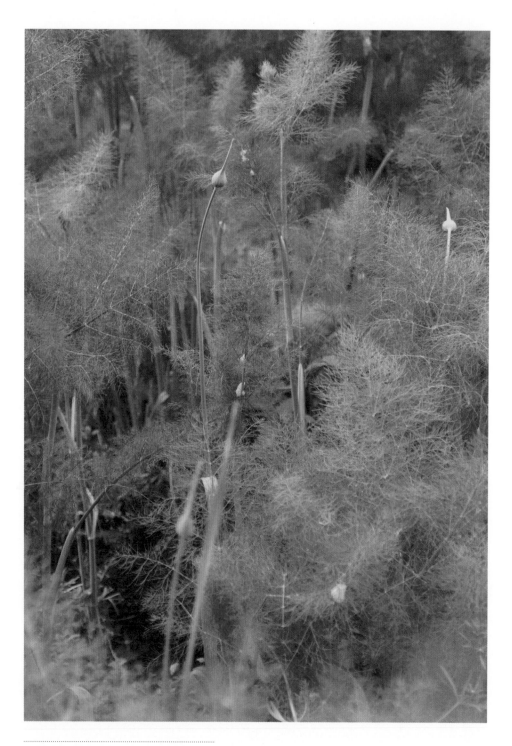

ABOVE: Fennel captured pre-bloom

RIGHT: Gingko in its delicate green glory

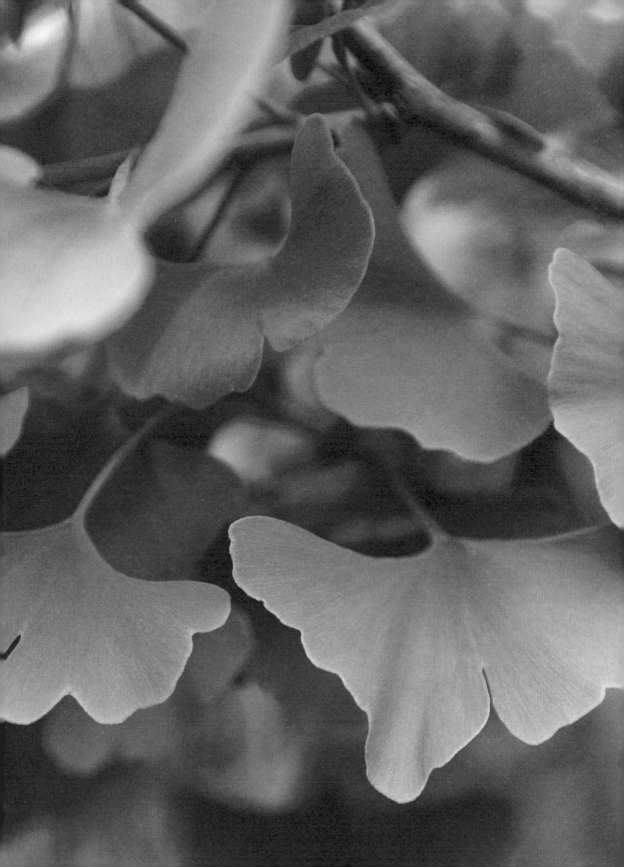

The Plant Path

The Plant Path

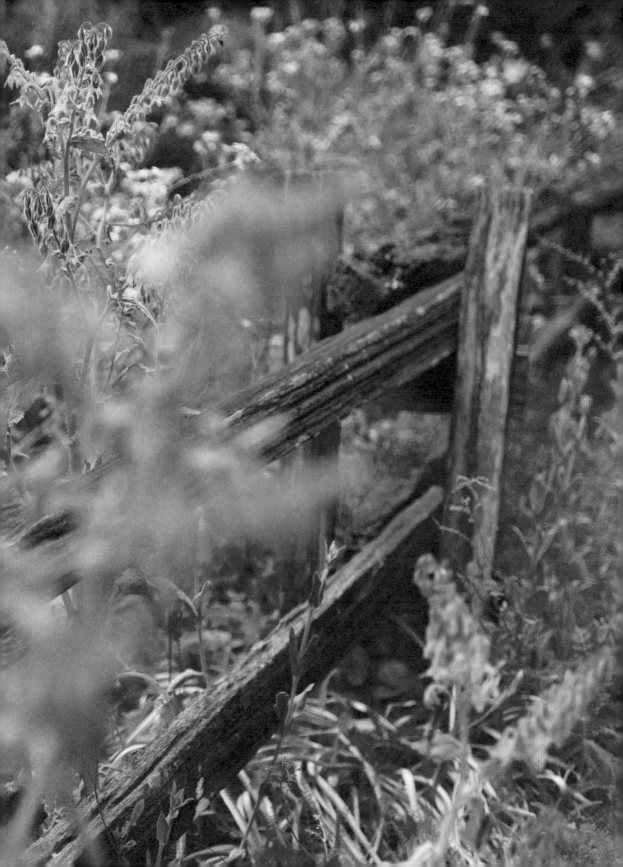

PLANTS FOR THE PEOPLE, PEOPLE FOR THE PLANTS

There is a much-loved belief among herbalists that the very plant you may need for your healing process is within your direct environment.

You might have forgotten your sense of belonging with the plants, your confidence to identify, wild-harvest, plant, nurture, grow, communicate. You might have forgotten your ability to bring forth healing. You might have misplaced your trust in your intuition. Well, brace yourself. This is the remembering.

We are waking up from a long slumber of disconnectedness. Remembering that we are made up of the same materials as nature. There is simply no separation. We the people are of the plants, and the plants are of the people.

Plants have been used by people in every way imaginable: for food, water, warmth, clothing, climate control and, of course, medicine. Before pharmaceuticals, only the plants existed as our allies for healing. Plants held the remedies, the healing, the relief. They have softened the fall, ceased the blood flow, eased the pain. They always have been, and always will be, the people's medicine.

Much of plant medicine begins with the traditional custodians of our lands, the Indigenous peoples. The first clans who walked the great plains learnt the language of the land for survival. Plants were viewed as guides and teachers. Our ancestors learnt a plant's story; they leaned in with their senses. They practised reciprocity with their environment; they listened to the earth and adjusted their rhythms accordingly. And then they left a legacy, preserving wisdom and passing on their knowledge – the process echoed in ancient cultures from one side of our world to the other. We must respect and hold gratitude for the traditional knowledge that has been passed down to us. There is a deep lineage within these realms of plant medicine. We do well to nod to the past as we harness the future.

Plant medicines are the embodiment of evolution: they evolve with us. Our complex human bodies have no ability to thrive without the plants. We are indebted to them. They are the air cleansers, the water regulators, the carbon dioxide transformers, the oxygenators, the bearers of the nutrients needed to sustain life. They are non-negotiable for our human experience. They are our lifeline.

In the magic of a wintry environment, the spruce trees stay green and brilliant, branches loaded with snow. When the echinacea, elder and goldenrod are sleeping, the spruce steps in to provide potent immune modulation and support, the elixir for the ailments of winter. The land is never against us; it works with us. This is the plant magic.

Back in the Middle Ages, the doctrine of signatures was created. This was a way to document learning and compile a database for herbal healing. This system of observation indicates how a plant's looks and habits relate to its impact on our bodies and beings. It speaks of messages signalled through a plant's appearance, via the colours and shapes of its structures, tastes, smells and the way in which it grows in its environment.

Through a plant's presentation we can learn how it may impact a body system, an organ or a condition, and even how it may affect an emotional state. The plant eyebright (*Euphrasia officinalis*) resembles a human eye and is commonly used for conditions of the eyes. Mullein (*Verbascum thapsus*) leaves have a soft and furry texture that bears a striking resemblance to our respiratory systems, and lo and behold, mullein is a classic lung tonic, wonderful for coughs, asthma support and bronchial recovery. Ginger (*Zingiber officinale*) looks much like the gnarled shape of a stomach, and we hail it for its ability to calm the belly.

We can thank the folk herbalism movement for preserving the doctrine of signatures: to this day it continues to be taught in the modern herbal class amid botany and pharmacology.

Take a plant like horsetail (*Equisetum arvense*), with its long tail-like structure and joint-like junctures along the stems and leaves. Horsetail is used to strengthen bones, to plump up joints, to fortify cartilage. This plant remedy has been in use for eons, and science confirms that horsetail is a powerhouse plant-based source of selenium, an essential trace mineral for bone health – just as those wise old folk herbalists said.

Do the plants activate our innate ability to heal, or is it the plant powers within that provide the compass and road map to healing? I believe it is both. I have witnessed tremendous transformations, gargantuan shifts and crystal-clear resolution of major health crises with the support of plant medicine. I commonly use the analogy that getting to the bottom of ill health is much like peeling a large onion: we peel back a layer to uncover another layer, and so forth. We eventually get to the centre, but not without patience and perseverance, and often with a few tears spilled.

Mostly, I work with chronic health conditions, from the gut to the thyroid, the skin, the uterus, and all in between. Many people have journeyed with their health challenges for a long time before they arrive at my clinic and turn to the plants for answers. Often they feel disenchanted and a little hopeless from their experience of the modern medical model. I am honoured to witness truly remarkable happenings daily in my clinic: stubborn skin infections clearing with echinacea (*Echinacea* spp.), goldenseal (*Hydrastis canadensis*) and garlic (*Allium sativum*); severe bloating and belly pain quietening with an aloe vera (*Aloe barbadensis*) and slippery elm (*Ulmus rubra*) concoction; cinnamon (*Cinnamomum verum*) and gymnema (*Gymnema sylvestre*) balancing blood sugar levels and easing sugar cravings; a long-missing menstrual cycle reappearing with chaste tree (*Vitex agnus-castus*) and peony (*Paeonia lactiflora*). Fenugreek (*Trigonella foenum-graecum*) and goat's rue (*Galega officinalis*) can support a new mamma struggling with breastmilk supply issues; valerian (*Valeriana officinalis*) can gently unlock tension and usher in a good night's sleep for the sleepless; turmeric (*Curcuma longa*) and devil's claw (*Harpagophytum procumbens*) can banish arthritic pain. Impressive, right?

One area I focus on in my practice is working alongside weary, exhausted, burnt-out people. So many people present with symptoms that are direct side effects of chronic stress. These side effects include exhaustion, anxiety, weight gain, sugar cravings, depression, hormonal imbalances ... and the list goes on. They are beyond on edge: their resilience is so low they have become completely intolerant of stress in any form. Their vitality tank is empty. This is the epidemic of our modern times.

My approach with these fatigued and frayed clients is to address every element visible, and to pay even closer attention to the invisible. I always, always, always employ adaptogenic herbs for these cases. Adaptogenic herbs are the superstar class of plant medicines that modulate the stress response in our bodies. They speak directly with the adrenal glands to impact the release of stress hormones and promote adaptation, recalibration and restoration. I have seen ashwagandha (*Withania somnifera*) wrap extremely deflated people in a warm embrace, restoring their light and fortifying their systems. Licorice (*Glycyrrhiza glabra*) has brought sweetness, balance and life back to the living. Rhodiola (*Rhodiola rosea*) awakens a deeper endurance and internal capacity to thrive, while schisandra (*Schisandra chinensis*) tonifies and increases resistance to what may come along. American ginseng (*Panax quinquefolius*) has woken the most exhausted souls I have ever seen. Adaptogens are essential for the weary – please remember this!

Plant medicine has taught me that there is no such thing as an impossible case. Years ago I helped a client with a severly weakened immune system. She was constantly getting ill, picking up every cold and bug, and being knocked around by them all. Alongside this, she was completely spent and weary; her day-to-day felt impossible to sustain. She was one of those incredibly health-conscious souls who ate clean and organic, drank spring water, exercised in a balanced manner and had a super-positive outlook. Why was she constantly so ill and exhausted?

I dug into her case and found a major underlying virus wreaking havoc on her health, piling pressure on her immune system and affecting her vitality. She was completely intolerant of anything in a capsule, sensitive to any vitamin. So we kept it simple. Working with stripped-back stand-out plant medicines to build immunity and vitality, I brought in one plant at a time, gently but surely, allowing the plants to meet her energy levels as she regained her footing. Echinacea (*Echinacea* spp.), elderberry (*Sambucus nigra*), thyme (*Thymus vulgaris*) and garlic (*Allium sativum*) all became a part of her every day. Ashwagandha (*Withania somnifera*) stepped in in full force to rebuild her energy levels. She got better, so much better. Once we uncover the roots of dis-ease, we can understand what is needed and the plant medicines become pillars to activate healing.

When you are ready to welcome them in, the plants can usher in profound change.

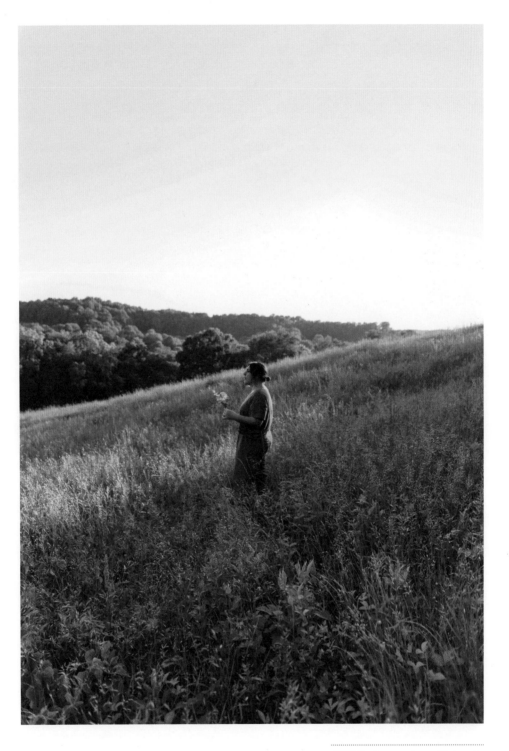

ABOVE: Communing with beauty
among fields of plant allies

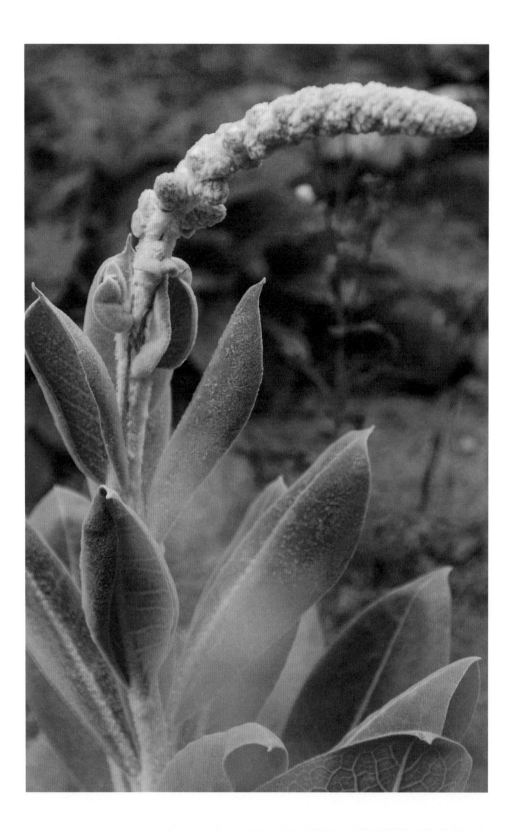

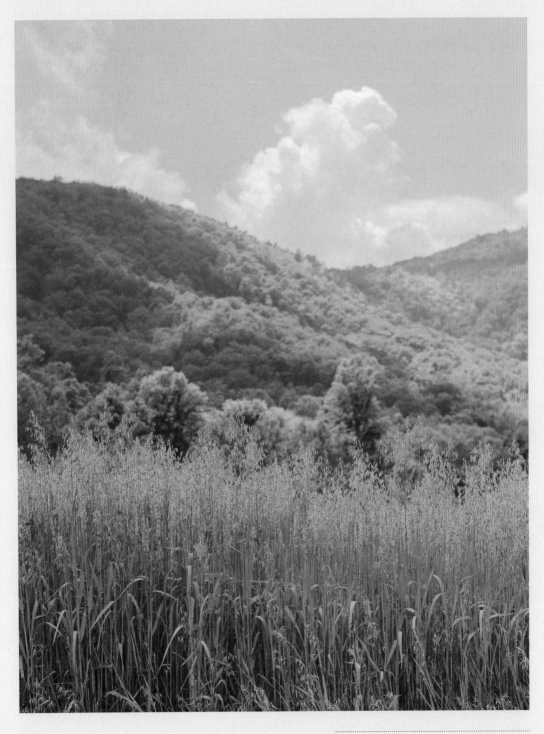

ABOVE: Oat fields standing tall and proud

LEFT: Mullein in early bloom

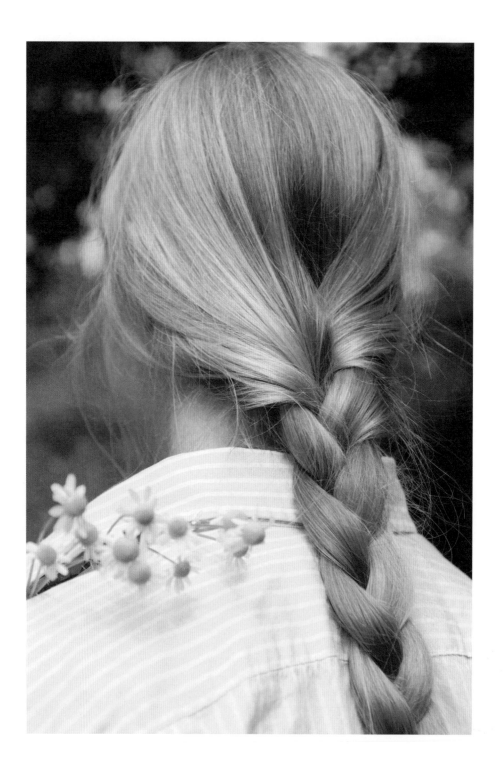

Plants for aches
Plants for anxiety
Plants for beauty
Plants for breastfeeding
Plants for burnout
Plants for children
Plants for coughs
Plants for depression
Plants for detoxification
Plants for digestion
Plants for eyesight
Plants for fatigue
Plants for fertility
Plants for focus
Plants for grief
Plants for grounding
Plants for heartbreak

Plants for immunity
Plants for infections
Plants for inflammation
Plants for libido
Plants for menstruation
Plants for metabolism
Plants for pain
Plants for peace
Plants for pregnancy
Plants for resilience
Plants for skin
Plants for sleep
Plants for sunburn
Plants for trauma
Plants for vitality
Plants for wounds

MIRRORING THE MESSAGES: THE BODY AND THE GARDEN

The greatest barometer is the body. Our bodies communicate to us with such clarity, we only have to take a moment to listen in. You may feel a headache, achy knees, an uncomfortable belly... this is the message. It takes a split second to ask yourself, 'How do I feel in my body today?'

We often overlook the hyper-surrealism of being human. In truth, if we honoured the complexity of our existence, we would likely not be very functional. We are walking miracles.

Our bodies offer us a sacred relationship, whether we partake in it or not. We are birthed so pure, but along the way we become influenced by the unrealistic standards society places on our bodies. We all ingest a cacophony of damaging messages and generally only begin to reclaim our truths as we age and recognise this distorted lens of perception. We often forget to hail the miracle of growing up, those gawky, awkward phases and the beauty of shapes and sizes ever-changing.

If only we lived in a utopian society where we were praised for the changes our bodies exhibit and met them with warm empathy and understanding. We would affirm a mamma's postnatal body recovering from the most spectacular act of all, teenagers' hormonal skin showing signs of coming into adulthood – a great initiation not without its growing pains. We would all dance with praise.

In an alternate reality we would ask daily, of our family, friends and peers, 'How are you feeling in your body today?' And they might answer, 'I feel a little tender in my heart' or 'A little scratchy in my throat. And you?'

In this parallel way of life, we would say warmly, 'Well, friend, I have the perfect ally for you. A little rose tea for your tender heart; an elderberry elixir for that scratchy throat.' It could be that simple. An offering of acknowledgement and support.

The beauty of this vision is that it can absolutely be your reality. Carving out a connection with plant medicine begins with your connection to self and comes straight from the heart.

Our greatest opportunity is to actually lean in and ask the question, 'How do I feel?' From this space, the remedies can pour in.

Within plant medicine there are many approaches, branches stemming ultimately from the same source. In the ethos of vitalist herbalism, everything is connected and driven by a vital force to grow, thrive and transform. The vitalist approach reflects that we are our own ecosystems in communion with the ecosystem of nature, and so the plants assist us to return to the balance we have forgotten. This is where plant medicine shines, mirroring our function as whole systems, with no separation between our physical, emotional, mental and spiritual bodies. All is connected.

Holism is related to vitalism, and the premise is anchored in approaching the body as a complete system, encouraging us to look not only to plants for medicine but also to food, water, body movement and rest to raise energy all round. Just as the soil needs to be tended for plant matter to grow deep roots, we need to tend to our own inner gardens.

There is no magic pill in herbalism; plant medicines do not work that way. They work with the forces of the body and spirit. They will not knock you out if you are in pain the way morphine will (morphine, by the way, was originally isolated from the opium poppy plant), but Californian poppy (*Eschscholzia californica*) will lull you into a space of soothed serenity when you are feeling agitated or sleepless. Plant medicines take their time, as does everything worthy.

We make a grave mistake if we begin to see plant medicine in an allopathic sense and try to bandaid symptoms. The call of any physical symptom is to address the root cause, the beginnings. Even in the realms of natural medicine, with its increasingly cerebral approach, we must remember not to mess with the perfection of nature; we don't need to overcomplicate it. This is whole plant medicine.

Plants are acts of kindness. Herbal medicine is kindness to the body, and approaching with kindness is a golden rule I implore you to follow as you deepen your relationship to plant medicine, and ultimately your interconnectedness with all living things.

Learning about the plants will provide you with an armoury of empowerment, for yourself and for those you hold dear, and is a powerful act of guardianship towards the earth. As we heal, the land heals in unison. We are activists reclaiming the right to know the medicine of self and soil.

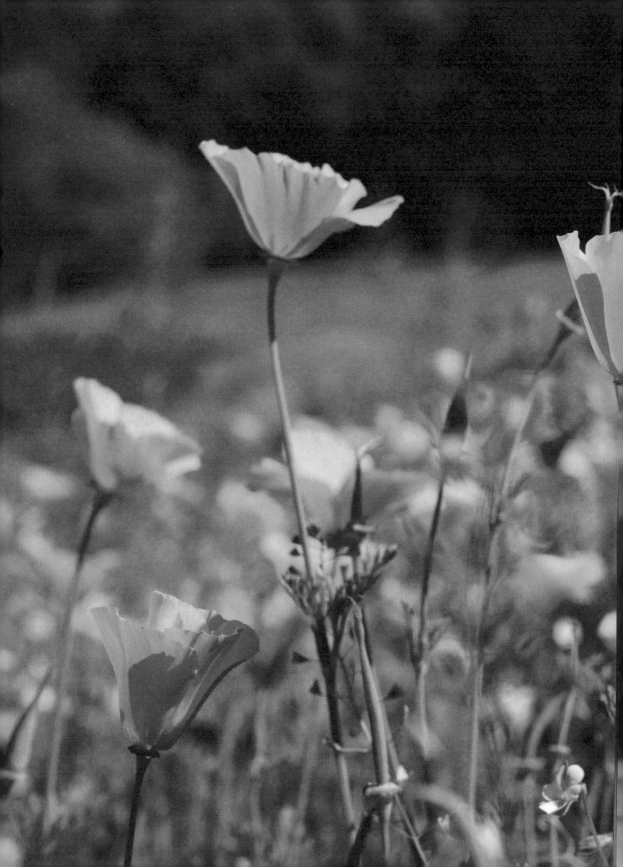

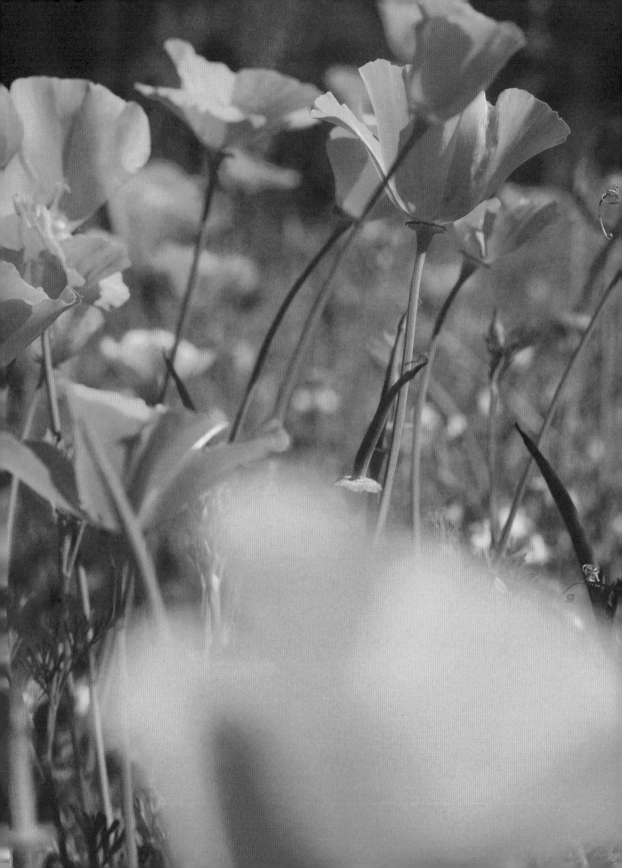

INTO THE WILD

Plant medicine is rooted in the wild places, the wild women; it was created in the wild, it proliferates in the wild.

Many of the plants profiled in this book are, in fact, classed as wild weeds, which may surprise you. Weeds are opportunistic: they can grow in the most inhospitable environments. They need no introduction; they just take up space, they adapt, they self-seed. They grow where gardeners wish they would not, often strangling the cultivated blooms we value so much. They are full of might and purpose.

Weeds have adapted with us, and if you pay close attention and understand their medicinal actions, you begin to understand why they persevere. They are packed full of nutrient-dense minerals and provide a source of wild food for living creatures; they offer nourishment to the seeker. They are resilient; they withstand critique and they don't give up. We can learn a whole lot from weeds. Let's reclaim their worth and listen to their wisdom.

Most people do not know that the elegant motherwort is considered a weed. She establishes herself in compost-rich, semi-shaded soil and grows much like her relative mint – they both proliferate with serious enthusiasm. Motherwort has a medicinal purpose, with the hint lying in her Latin name, *Leonurus cardiaca*, which translates to 'the lion heart'. She has an affinity for the cardiovascular system – our red, beating hearts. She holds the energy of the mother, invoking nourishment and peace, balancing menstrual cycles and easing an anxious, racing heartbeat. Can you see why she grows so abundantly and freely? It is because the lion's heart is needed. This is a plant for our times. May the weedy wonders of her seed spread and find their way matured and blooming into our homes and hearts.

Dandelion, chickweed, gotu kola, red clover, mugwort, cleavers, fennel, nettle, plantain, milk thistle, evening primrose, mullein… the list goes on. These valued plant medicines are all common weeds.

Take St John's wort (*Hypericum perforatum*), for instance. This easy-to-come-by weed grows in many locations worldwide. There is little concern about overharvesting, and many farmers would gladly open their fields for you to pick the flower when blooming, as it can be an invasive plant. When consumed in high amounts, St John's wort can cause photosensitivity in grazing cattle and sheep, due to the active constituent hypericin. There are hundreds of species of hypericum, but once you get to know this plant, you will be certain of its identity. St John's wort is a leggy, woody-based plant growing to 60–90 centimetres (2–3 feet) high, whose abundant yellow flower heads hit full bloom in summertime. It is a sight to behold – gangs of cheerful, sunny fleurs saluting the sun in open fields and along roadsides.

Another stellar example of a weedy wonder-plant is mullein (*Verbascum thapsus*). Not at all subtle, this bold biennial stands proudly erect, often growing beyond 2 metres (6½ feet) tall. It is an impressive plant, with large, oval-shaped, pale-green, silver-tinted leaves that feel like the fuzziest soft velvet. In the second year of its life cycle, a strong stalk strikes upwards, bearing clusters of brilliant yellow five-petalled flowers. Commonly referred to as a wayside weed, mullein grows in all sorts of conditions. You may see it alongside sandy sloping hills or highways, in open paddocks or rocky terrain. It loves to live in disturbed habitats and also enjoys being by the water. Leaves are best collected in the first year of the plant's life, when the vital force of the plant is condensed in the lower sections. As the plant sends up its stalk, the force focuses on the potency of the flowers. These flowers will pop throughout the summer months, when the yellow heads are collected for medicine making. After a mullein plant has lived its life, a new incarnation will pop up very close by, in a cyclical nature.

These two plants are medicinal superstars, growing plentifully and sustainably in many naturescapes.

Regardless of where in the world you are located, there will be medicinal weeds right in your backyard, in the urban alley, on the edges of the football field, in the lush meadows.

This is the foundation of bioregional herbalism, the practice of approaching the land within reach for medicine, as there are always remedies to be found in our immediate environment. We therefore cultivate a sincere connection to and coexistence with the nature we live among. The medicinal bounty may vary in form from place to place, but trust me, it is never too far away when you hear the wildcrafting call.

Wildcrafting is the practice of collecting uncultivated plants from their natural habitat, plants that grow wild and free without any intervention. This is foraging at its very best; it demands only respect, attuned wits, a pair of pruners, capable hands and a basket. Wildcrafting is essentially the practice of deepening a connection with the land, in which you become a guardian for regeneration and care.

What is important with wildcrafting and wild harvesting is that you must be beyond sure of the plant you are picking. Be completely certain of its identity. To help with this, I have provided some wonderful literature and guides in the resource section on page 204 that will get you on the way to becoming a wildcrafting pro. Many plants are very easy to identify, just like mullein, but others, like yarrow (*Achillea millefolium*), can easily be confused with other plants. Best to practise due diligence!

There is a strong code of ethics to wildcrafting that we all must follow to ensure the longevity of medicinal ecosystems.

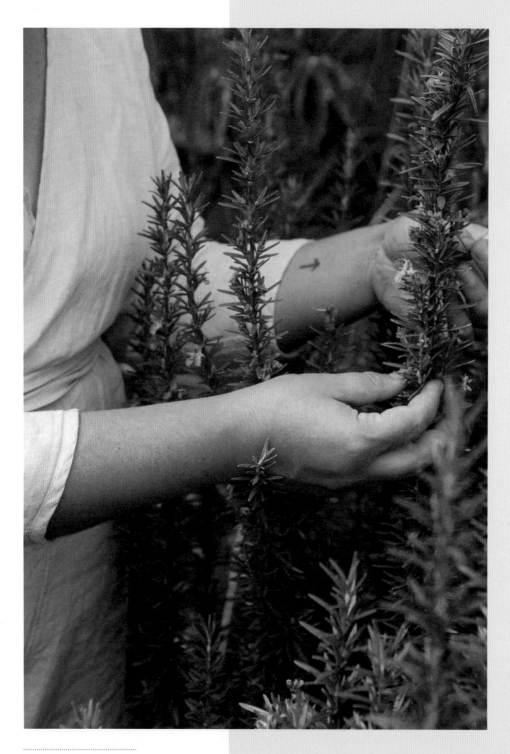

ABOVE: Hardy and wise
rosemary in flower

WILDCRAFTING GOLDEN RULES

Wild harvesting must be done well away from busy roads, highways, agricultural farmland and industrial areas. Thirty to 60 metres (100–200 feet) away from any utilised roads is a good rule of thumb.

....

+ If there is any chance of chemical spray or contamination, most definitely avoid the area.

+ Be sure to avoid trespassing on private land: not everywhere is open to wildcrafting visitors.

+ Ensure you are safe; the plants want that for you.

+ Steer clear of any endangered plant species; we need them to regain their footing, so give them space.

+ Be sure to harvest in the correct season for the plant.

+ Harvest in the cooler parts of the day, when possible. This causes less stress for the plant, and your plant material will retain its vibrancy better than if picked in full heat.

+ Commune with the plants, ask for permission, give thanks to the plants.

+ Positively identify the plant without a doubt before harvesting. Safety is our priority.

+ Go for middle-growth areas, not the biggest or smallest plants.

+ Aim to harvest the top third of the plant (most plant collection calls for flowering tops, foliage, stems, branches). Do not take the whole plant or roots if it can be avoided. It is essential to leave the seeds behind for future yield from where the plant was retrieved.

+ Only take what is needed: there is no need to overharvest as this is detrimental to plant populations. Think of harvesting one out of every five plants growing in the area you are picking from.

+ Step gently. Leave the space a little more loved than you found it: for example, pick up any garbage. Imagine you are in your great-aunt's house, and you are on your best behaviour!

....

If we follow these steps, we can gain so much gold from the experience of foraging wild plant medicines. The greatest place to begin, though, for any novice or expert, is in your very own backyard. This is where the wild weedy ones grow, uncomplicated and eager to assist.

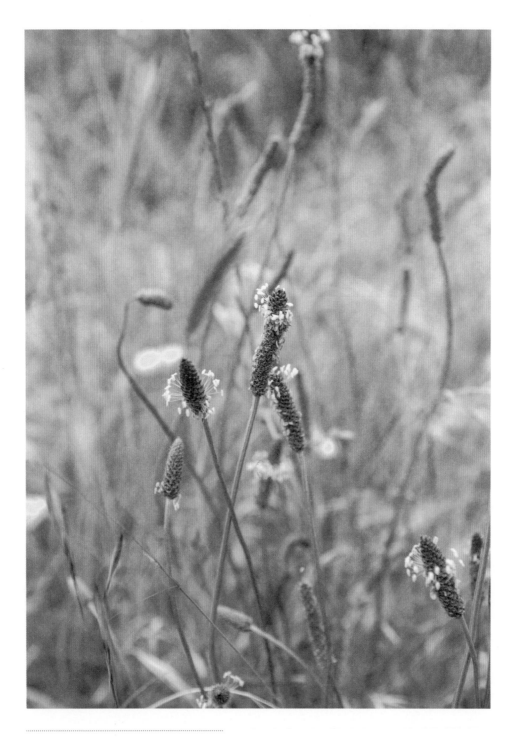

ABOVE: Ribwort plantain, an abundant
wild weed, swaying in the breeze

RIGHT: Nasturtiums in full spring blossom

HOW TO USE PARTS 2 AND 3

In this book I'm working from a core group of herbal 'hero plants'. Before you dive into learning the plants and making plant medicines, please know that this is doable for everyone. You come from different backgrounds and live all over this great globe, with different needs and rhythms. Your allies, the plants, are everywhere and offer ways to work with them that are completely universal.

Just a couple of key points to remind you that you have indeed got this!

+ You do not need to be a wildcrafter or a professional gardener to get to know plant medicine. You begin gently where you are planted – it is truly that simple. Many online and local stores offer prepared dried herbs, making it incredibly easy to find the ingredients you seek.

+ You do not need to source only organic herbs, but I would strongly suggest you ensure they are chemical free and sourced ethically. These are conscious decisions we make when possible that have a great impact on farmers, small growers, the environment and ultimately our health.

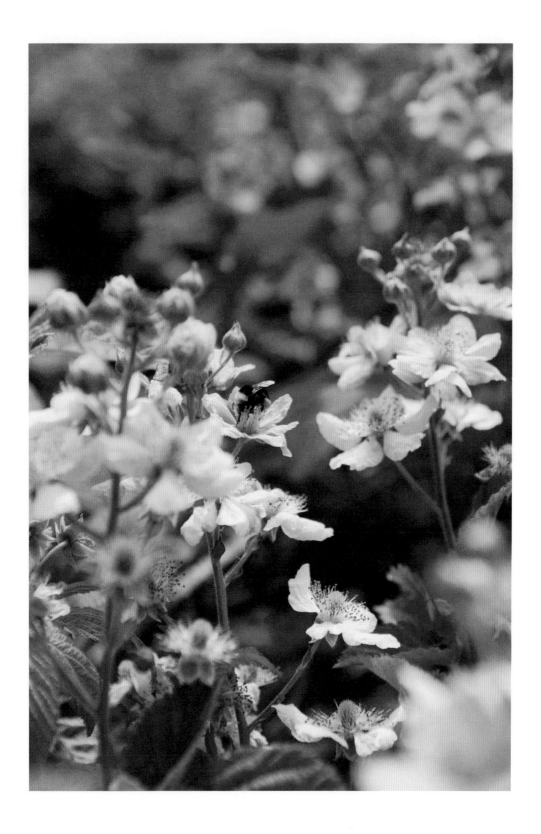

The Wild Healers

The Wild Healers

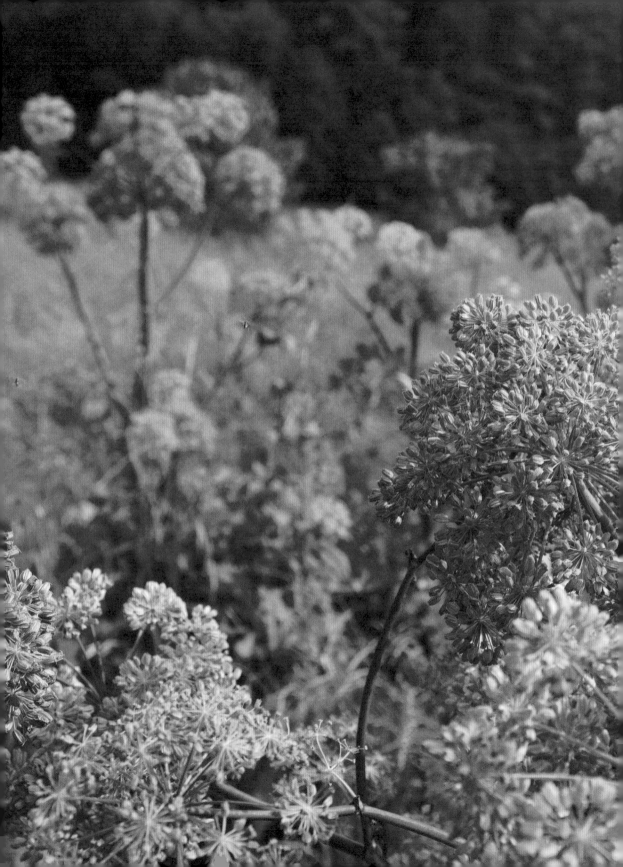

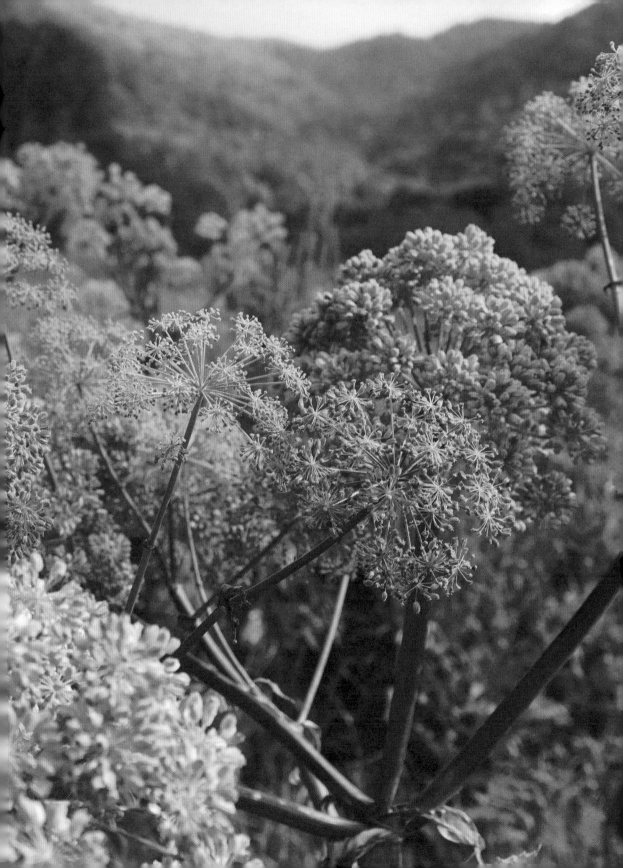

THE PLANT MEDICINE PANTRY

Building a home apothecary can be a little daunting. Where to begin?

Start by filling your shelves with the berries, leaves, flowers, buds, barks, roots and rhizomes that call you. There really isn't much better than a bountiful dispensary.

STORING YOUR HERBALS

The shelf life of dried herbs varies, so employ your senses to check their freshness. How they smell, taste and appear is the best way to gauge their viability and medicinal life force. The best way to store your herbals is in airtight, sealed glass jars that can be kept well away from direct light – in a cool, dark cupboard is ideal. We herbalists generally prefer to bottle our dried herbs, tinctures, salves and creams in amber-toned glass to keep them unspoilt and extra fresh.

FRESH OR DRIED PLANTS?

You cannot beat a fresh plant harvest, so where possible, of course, choose fresh! However, there can be limitations to working with fresh plant material. A fresh plant medicine needs to be used up quick smart – for example, in a poultice – whereas a dried plant preparation, such as a dried-root tea blend, can be safely stored for long periods of time. Dried plants are much easier to access, dodging the seasonal limitations of fresh plants, and are concentrated in potency. Fresh plants are a little trickier and susceptible to rancidity, especially in oil infusions, although there are some exceptions. This is why I generally suggest using dried herbs in the recipes to come.

   If you are using fresh herbs in these recipes, be sure to double the recommended amount in replacement of the dried herbs. Also, you can totally blend fresh and dry herbs – just be sure to use the plant potion immediately.

THE IMPORTANCE OF THE SOURCE

Non-organically grown plants are sprayed with many potentially harmful chemicals; when steeped in a small amount of water, such as in a tea, the chemical residue becomes condensed. It is highly advisable to source organically grown plant material from reputable growers and stores. Where possible, opt for locally grown plants: there is extra synergy working with plants in tune with the land you stand on. Growing your own plant medicines can be incredibly rewarding, and an opportunity to get to know the plants intimately, or head into the wilds for a forage, but please remember to follow the foraging guidelines outlined on page 35.

A NOTE ON INGREDIENTS

All of the wild healer recipes are based on the forty plant personalities you will meet in the pages to come. However, for the sake of your tastebuds, I have added a few extra elements to round out flavour and palatability, because as we all know (or you will soon find out), not all plant medicines are easy on the senses!

STERILISING 1, 2, 3

Many of the recipes call for you to mix and/or store your plant-powered potions in sterilised jars or bottles. This ensures that any harmful bacteria, yeasts or fungi are banished from the vessels before you fill them with your finished remedies. The two methods I use, listed below, are simple. And a little extra tip: try to sterilise your glass vessels as close as possible to bottling time.

Stovetop: Fill a large saucepan with cold water and submerge the jars and lids in the pot. Bring to a full boil, then reduce the heat to medium and keep at a consistent boil for 10 minutes. Remove the sterilised containers and lids, and allow them to air-dry.

Dishwasher: Use the hottest cycle to sterilise your vessels. When complete, remove the jars and lids, and allow them to air-dry completely.

A FRIENDLY CAUTION

Most importantly, please refer to the plant profiles in Part 3 to really get to know the essence and therapeutic story of the plants. Many of the blends following are cautioned or contraindicated for use during pregnancy and lactation, so please always practise diligence in researching which plants are in alignment with the cycle you are currently in.

Also, please understand that not all herbal medicines are indicated for use with infants and children; some are far too strong energetically and medicinally. Always err on the side of caution and consult a herbalist or naturopathic practitioner when in doubt.

DOSING THE WILD HEALERS

Symptoms offer us a portal and are constantly giving us clues to how we can dig deep for the roots of dis-ease. Meeting the energetics of the symptom is key! If there is a chronic health condition that has been with you for a long period of time – an illness or long-term allergy, for example – the plant medicines need to be taken for longer periods, to go deeper into the old stories the body has been expressing. If there is more of an acute presentation – a viral cold, a flu, a headache – it is best to dose the plant medicine frequently to calm the symptomatic intensity and offer support.

Be mindful that dosages for infants and children vary greatly from an adult dose; little ones need far less!

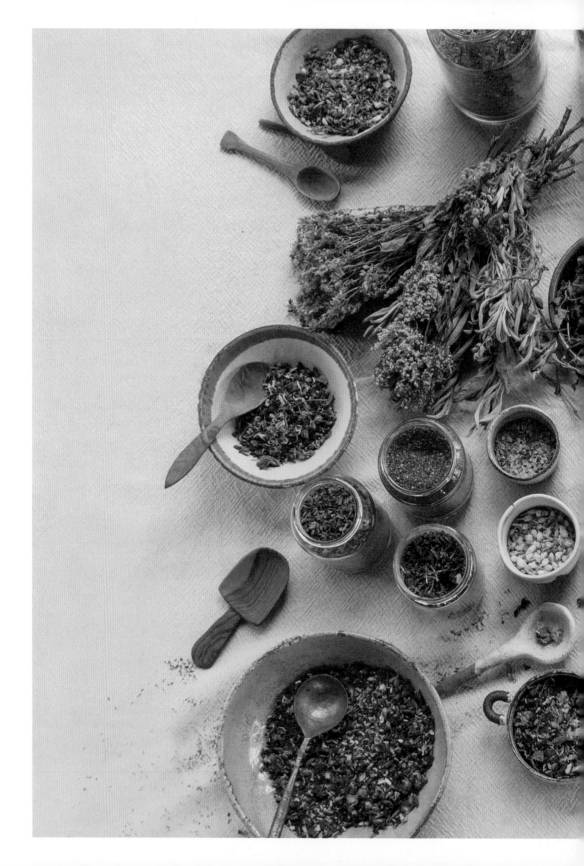

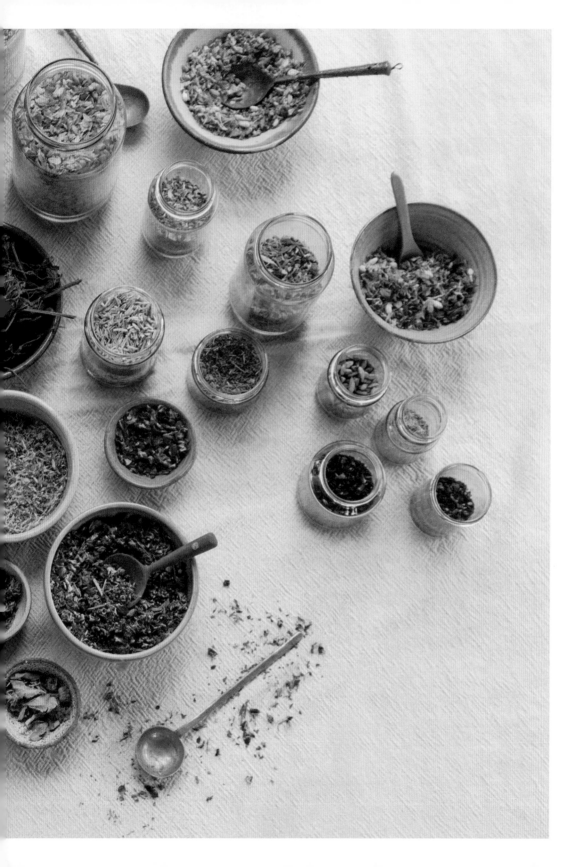

TEAS, INFUSIONS, DECOCTIONS, SUN BREWS

Often the easiest approach is the most potent.

Teas, infusions, decoctions and sun brews have been in use for as long as plants and people have been kin, and are four of the most accessible ways to work with plants, dried or fresh.

Essentially, infusions, decoctions and sun brews follow the principles of tea, but they are amplified in the medicinal sense.

Medicinal teas are made by steeping the plant material in boiling water for a quick 10–20 minutes. Follow with a simple strain and sip mindfully.

An infusion involves a longer steeping in boiling water, for a gentle extraction and activation of the plant material. It is best used for the softer aerial parts of a plant – think flowers, leaves, buds and berries. Bear in mind that there are some plants that prefer a cold-water infusion as their delicate properties are sensitive to heat. Infusions extract the volatile oils, vitamins and precious enzymes of medicinal plants, so be sure to cover the infusing concoction to trap all of these beneficial elements. Infusions can be 20–30 minute brews or left for 4–12 hours to deepen the medicinal impact.

A decoction is used more for the woody parts of plants – think roots, rhizomes, seeds, twigs, bark – which require more time and amplified heat to liberate the medicinal constituents. A decoction calls for a slow, covered boil, around 20–40 minutes.

A sun brew is simply an infusion made by combining dried or fresh herbs with filtered water, sealing and popping out in the sun to brew for a day.

A golden principle of medicinal teas, infusions, decoctions and sun brews is that they are best used straight away. As water is their base, there is no preservative present and we want to avoid any mould formation. However, infusions can be kept for up to 24 hours; sun brews and decoctions can be refrigerated and will stay active for around 48 hours.

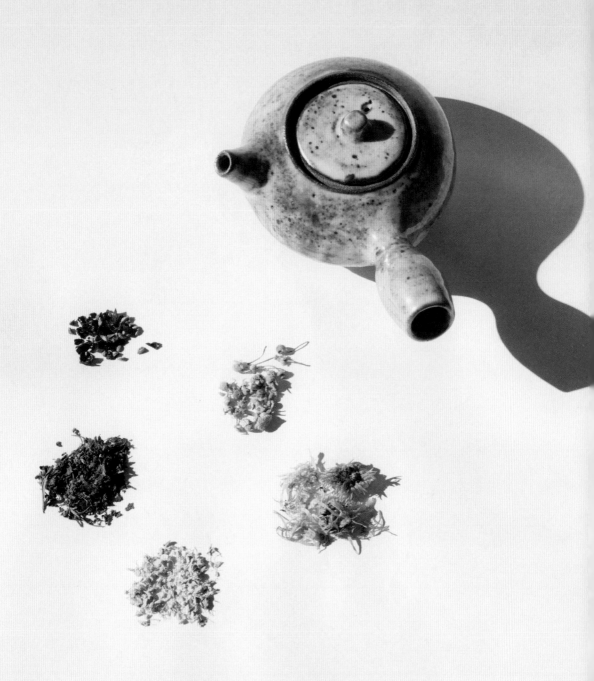

A GUIDE TO BREWING MEDICINAL PLANTS

HERBAL TEAS
Pour boiling water over the dried or fresh herbs and steep for 10–20 minutes. Strain out the plant material with a fine-mesh sieve, and enjoy.

INFUSIONS
Add the plant material to a heatproof mason jar, fill with boiling water and infuse for 3–4 hours minimum, or leave overnight to deepen the strength. Simply strain out the herbs with a fine-mesh sieve and sip throughout the day. Infusions make a perfect iced tea; however, if you desire a little warmth, you can gently heat on the stove.

DECOCTIONS
Simply add your hardy herbs to a saucepan with water, and bring to a boil. Allow the concoction to simmer for at least 20–30 minutes, then strain and enjoy!

SUN BREWS
Spoon the herbal blend of your choice into a glass jar, generally filling around half the jar with fresh plant material or a quarter of the jar with dried plants. Fill to the brim with cool water, pop on a muslin top or a lid to keep the bugs away, and leave out in a sunny spot to imbue the brew with warmth.

MEASURING THE MEDICINALS
The recipes ahead are measured in parts. This is a clear and flexible way to outline a formula and allows you to be interpretive with your units of measurement. For instance, if the recipe calls for one part peppermint, this may equal 1 cup, 1 tablespoon or 1 teaspoon of peppermint. The important rule is to keep the ratios of the recipe the same, and just adjust your method of measuring! For a medium pot of tea, use a base of 2 cups of water for a regular-strength herbal brew in all of the following recipes.

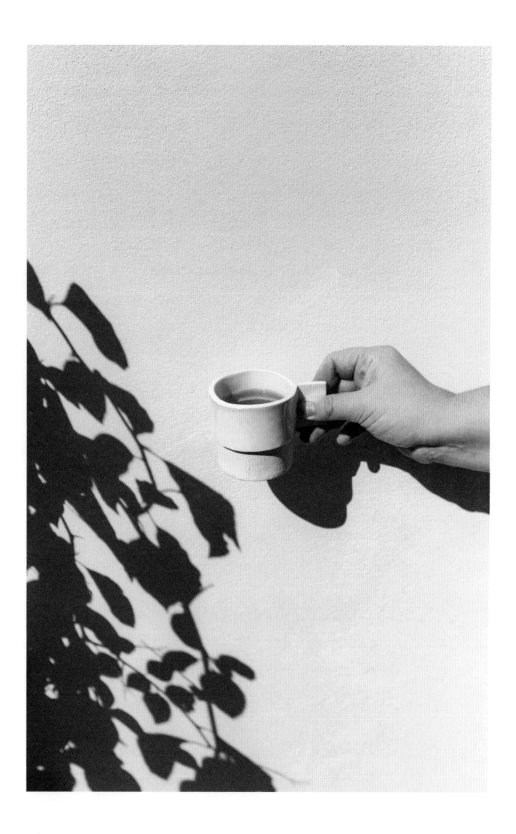

IMMUNITY

Our bodies commonly speak to us with symptoms to convey a message – it may be a quiet conversation or a deafening directive. Symptoms signal the need for rest, to rein it in, to ease the pace. The herbal blends here are wonderful for an active cold or flu. To elevate the medicinal magic, create an overnight infusion of your chosen blend. Be sure to increase the frequency of dosing up to 2–6 cups daily if you have been struck with the low-immunity stick! To support immunity generally, weave these wild healers into your daily rituals.

Bronchial buster

A potent mix for the sinuses, persistent coughs, asthma and bacterial infections. These common kitchen herbs have strong antiviral, antibacterial and warming properties. Lighten the flavour with a squeeze of fresh lemon juice or some raw honey.

2 parts thyme
2 parts oregano
2 parts rosemary
1 part cinnamon chips

Best prepared as a tea

Bye-bye flu

This power-packed combination of immune tonics and lymphatic-loving herbals works to shift an active flu and support an overburdened immune system. Brew strongly, and be sure to sip frequently to alleviate symptoms.

3 parts cleavers leaf/stem/flowers
2 parts calendula flowers
2 parts echinacea root/leaf/flowers
2 parts elderflowers
1 part cinnamon chips
1 part elderberries
1 part orange peel, fresh or dried
½ part lemon balm

Best prepared as a tea or infusion

Defender

This is a beautifully supportive tea, high in immune-enhancing herbs and vitamin C. It can be drunk daily to fortify immunity, or utilised to combat the common cold. I like to add a touch of manuka honey when the tea cools to supercharge the immune-enhancing effects.

2 parts elderberries
2 parts echinacea root/flowers/leaf
1 part rosehips
½ part ginger pieces
½ part cinnamon chips
manuka honey (optional)

Best prepared as a tea or infusion

Deep breath

The demulcent actions of the herbs in this blend work together to combat a hoarse, sore throat and soothe relentless coughs, supporting the lungs and gently sedating any upper-respiratory irritation or spasms. As this brew cools, add an optional dollop of medicinal manuka honey.

3 parts mullein leaf
1 part sage
1 part thyme
½ part licorice root
manuka honey (optional)

Best prepared as a tea or infusion

Y.E.P.

Yarrow, elder and peppermint is a classic botanical blend of synergistic herbs. It has a light flavour with minty, sweet tones, and will break up respiratory catarrh and congestion, and reduce inflammation associated with an active immune bug. Y.E.P. tea has long been used to reduce fever, alongside relieving the symptoms and duration of colds and flus. Do your best to drink this tea as hot as possible – the heat is thought to encourage the breaking of a fever.

1 part yarrow leaf
1 part elderberries
1 part peppermint

Best prepared as a tea or infusion

DIGESTION

The gut is a clear barometer of health. Our digestive systems and emotions interact in call and response; we are simply wired that way. Stress wreaks havoc on our sensitive bellies, and physical symptoms prove this super-duper clearly, with bloating, nausea, changeable bowel habits, excess gas and reflux all common expressions of a stressed system. Our guts are responsible for so many major functions: absorbing nutrients, regulating immunity and hormones, eliminating waste, fending off pathogens, producing serotonin, supporting the microbiota, and a gazillion other duties. It makes sense that a harmonious digestive system sets us up for good health. The gut is like a garden: we must tend the soil, chase away the pests and sow the seeds so that we may flourish wildly.

Mover and a shaker

A blend for a slow-moving bowel, full of encouraging herbs to promote motion and ease the uncomfortable symptoms associated with a bunged-up belly!

2 parts dandelion root
1½ parts fennel seed
1½ parts cinnamon chips
¼ part licorice root

Best prepared as a decoction

Sweet relief

For a bloated, gas-filled belly, to usher in comfort and relief. A lovely after-dinner blend to aid digestion while preparing the body for a good night's sleep.

2 parts chamomile flowers
2 parts peppermint
1 part licorice root
1 part rosehips
1 part fennel seed
¼ part ginger pieces

Best prepared as a tea or infusion

Bunch of bitters

Brace yourself to awaken your digestive system! Simply brew this blend and sip 20 minutes before a meal. Bitters stimulate beneficial digestive juices, which are essential to break down food and maintain a happy belly!

1½ parts cinnamon chips
1 part dandelion root
1 part motherwort leaf/flowers

Best prepared as a decoction

Miracle worker

For those dire times when your belly is letting everything go, ferociously. To combat loose stools and diarrhoea, this highly astringent, calming blend will help regulate the bowel so you can spend far less time on the loo.

1 part yarrow leaf
1 part raspberry leaf
1 part chamomile flowers

Best prepared as a tea or infusion

Bugs be gone

Be aware: this combo is not for the faint-hearted! A bitter antimicrobial combo, with minty tones to settle and soften the edges. Wonderful for candida, intestinal worms and parasitic overgrowths.

3 parts peppermint
2 parts thyme
2 parts chickweed
1½ parts sage
1 part oregano
½ part wormwood flowers/leaf

Best prepared as a tea

VITALITY

We hold a bonfire of vitality within, yet sometimes the flames dwindle; the small embers may still crackle, but there is no blaze to be seen. The keeper of our life force, our vitality, suffers when it is underfed, and the need to revitalise and restore it is often overlooked. In our speedy modern day, where burnout is high, and there are anxiety, depression and health crises aplenty, it is essential to dip our cups into the well of regeneration and sacred self-care. The plants have an incredible way of raising vitality; they have an innate ability to restore deficient and depleted energy, rehabilitating and reinstating our inner glow.

....

Restorer

A powerful quartet to decompress and revitalise the adrenal glands, aiding our cortisol response and refuelling the tank. Much like a hug in a cup, this is the blend to employ when reserves are low and to combat exhaustion.

3 parts ashwagandha root
2 parts gotu kola leaf
2 parts lemon balm
1 part licorice root

Best prepared as a tea or infusion

....

Peacemaker

A gentle nervine-laden blend to welcome in harmony and serenity, quieten anxiety and calm a busy brain with the soothing forces of plant magic.

2 parts passionflower
2 parts oat straw
1 part chamomile flowers
½ part rosehips

Best prepared as a tea or infusion

Lighten the load

Melt away stress and tame tension, lightening your load with the uplifting and relaxing effects of the sacred tulsi, zen master passionflower, hypnotic lavender and wise sage.

3 parts tulsi
2 parts passionflower
1 part lavender flowers
½ part sage leaf

Best prepared as a tea or infusion

Bright light

Lifting the fog and easing the blues, the sunshine chalice, St John's wort, permeates the spirit with a sense of lightness, paving the way for light to shine in.

3 parts St John's wort flowers/leaf/stem
3 parts lemon balm
2 parts oat straw

Best prepared as a tea or infusion

Heart ease

For the heavy-hearted, for melancholia, for the grief-struck. Motherwort, the heart healer, offers refuge, while the petals of the rose bring the colour back into your heart. The added spices lift the mind and clear the spirit.

2 parts motherwort leaf/flowers
2 parts rose petals
2 parts cinnamon chips
1 part cardamom pods

Best prepared as a tea or infusion

The daily multi

The essential herbal multivitamin, this supercharged mix contains a wealth of minerals and vitamins for a daily nutritional boost. High in vitamin C, iron, calcium, B vitamins and much more, this is best made as a large infusion to be sipped throughout the day. Also makes a delicious iced tea!

3 parts raspberry leaf
2 parts red clover flowers
1½ parts nettle leaf
1 part oat straw
1 part peppermint
1 part goji berries
½ part rosehips

Best prepared as an overnight infusion

Cloud nine

A heavenly blend to raise energy levels, stimulate high vibes and eradicate dullness of the mind, body and spirit.

3 parts yarrow leaf
2 parts tulsi leaf
1 part yarrow flowers
1 part peppermint
1 part rose petals

Best prepared as a tea or infusion

Wise woman

For the wonder women, a crisp green garden of goodness! This tonifying combination fortifies the yin forces within, bringing gentle support to the adrenal glands, balancing hormones and grounding the nervous system.

2 parts lemon balm
2 parts nettle leaf
1 part motherwort leaf/flowers
1 part mugwort leaf/flowers
1 part sage
½ part dried lemon peel

Best prepared as a tea or infusion

Warmth of the sun

Rich in nutritive herbs and antioxidants, this nourishing tea is best brewed in the glory of the sunshine. Adding raw honey to taste when the tea is ready rounds out the tang and makes this one easy-to-drink tonic!

3 parts raspberry leaf
2 parts red clover flower
½ part dried orange peel
½ part rosehips
½ part hibiscus flowers
honey (optional)

Best prepared as a sun brew or long infusion

The perfect pair

The simplest and mightiest duo. The combination of nettle leaf and oat straw as a long infusion is quite legendary. Deeply replenishing, with a cocktail of minerals and vitamins, these two plant wizards raise vitality and restore tired, frazzled and depleted folk. Extra delicious with a touch of sweetener, this earthy blend pairs well with either raw honey or blackstrap molasses for an extra mineral-rich dose!

1 part nettle leaf
1 part oat straw

Best prepared as a long infusion

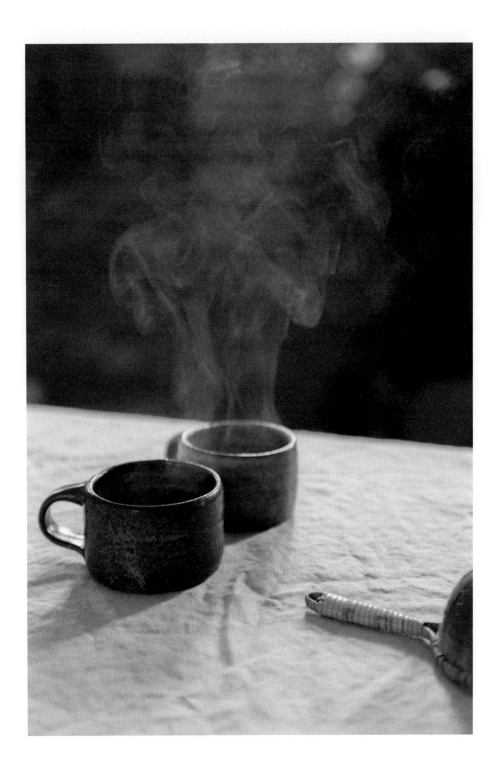

CLEANSE

Our bodies have a wise way of detoxifying naturally through our channels of elimination. When these channels become sluggish and overloaded due to stress, poor dietary choices, alcohol, lack of sleep and environmental burdens, we can often feel a little toxic. Physical symptoms may flare: frequent aches and pains, breakouts, elevated exhaustion...

Fortifying the energy of our elimination systems to enhance cleansing and usher in purification is essential. Luckily we have an abundance of hero herbals to reach out to when we need backup to come on in and shake things up!

Root to bloom

There is nothing more grounding than sipping on roots and rhizomes. This earthy blend will aid the liver and gall bladder to do their work with extra efficiency, clearing out stagnancy and encouraging detoxifying flow.

1 part dandelion root
½ part turmeric rhizome
¼ part ginger pieces

Best prepared as a decoction

The restorative cleanse

A combination to clear an overheated liver and gently cleanse the lymphatic system, while tonifying the kidneys and adrenal glands. Rooibos and hibiscus elevate the taste and offer their high antioxidant content to this nourishing blend.

3 parts rooibos
2 parts nettle leaf
1 part dandelion root
1 part oat straw
½ part hibiscus flowers

Best prepared as a tea or infusion

Weeded wonder chai

A way to keep chai in your life, minus the caffeine! The wild weed nettle anchors the blend, offering her nutrient-dense leaf high in vitamins and minerals. Coupled with a tribe of beneficial spices to warm and uplift the spirit, this is the perfect antidote to sluggishness.

2 parts nettle leaf
½ part cinnamon chips
½ part ginger pieces
½ part cardamom pods
½ part star anise
¼ part cloves
¼ part whole peppercorns

Best prepared as a combination of overnight infusion of the nettle leaf and decoction of all other parts

Heat tamer

An anti-inflammatory, antioxidant-rich blend to calm the overactive heat within, particularly achy and inflamed joints. Turmeric and black pepper join harmoniously to enhance bioavailability, while the sweet, warm, citrusy tones bring deliciousness.

2 parts rooibos
2 parts turmeric rhizome
2 parts cinnamon chips
1 part rosehips
¼ part dried orange peel
¼ part dried lemon peel
¼ part whole peppercorns
¼ part ginger pieces

Best prepared as a decoction

Inner glow

A blend to activate the shine within, perfect for boosting the lymphatic system to brighten dull skin, or ease a congested complexion.

1½ parts red clover flowers
1 part rooibos
1 part calendula
1 part cleavers leaf/stem/flowers
1 part mullein leaf
1 part echinacea root/flowers/leaf
½ part ginger pieces

Best prepared as a tea or infusion

SLEEP

The most essential healing you can give to your body is sweet, restful sleep. Evolution dictates that we generally need eight hours of sleep per night; this is one area that needs no biohacking! Often elusive, sleep is something we chase and when we can't catch it, we quickly begin to feel the effects. Poor sleep creates all sorts of chaos for our body, mind and spirit. Practising sleep hygiene, turning down the noise of the day and welcoming in the calm energy of the evening, is essential. The perfect night-time ritual to wind down with is a cup of herbal comfort ushering in deep rest and renewal.

Sweet dreams

A gentle supportive trio to soothe the nervous system and welcome in a zen state of mind, heart and spirit. Full of calming nervines, perfect to take the edge off and yield to the yin energy of the evening.

2 parts oat straw
2 parts lemon balm
1 part chamomile flowers

Best prepared as a tea or infusion

Deep slumber

The antidote to light, restless sleep, this synergistic combo opens up the gateway for peaceful rest and is far more efficient than counting sheep. Brew this one strong and mighty for maximum medicinal power.

2 parts passionflower
2 parts lemon balm
1 part valerian root

Best prepared as a tea or infusion

Floral lullaby

Let the blooms sing a sweet song of soothing serenity to lull you into the dream realm. There really is nothing better than sipping on flowers, and this mix is full of them!

3 parts passionflower
1½ parts chamomile flowers
1 part Californian poppy flowers/leaf/stem
½ part lavender flowers

Best prepared as a tea or infusion

Into the mystic

An activator of the higher planes, this blend speaks to the energy centres of the third eye and crown chakra, accessing intuition and psychic abilities. If you feel you are experiencing lacklustre dreams, this blend will take you deep into the dream sphere.

2 parts tulsi leaf
2 parts gotu kola leaf
1 part chamomile flowers
1 part dried orange peel
½ part mugwort leaf/flowers

Best prepared as a tea or infusion

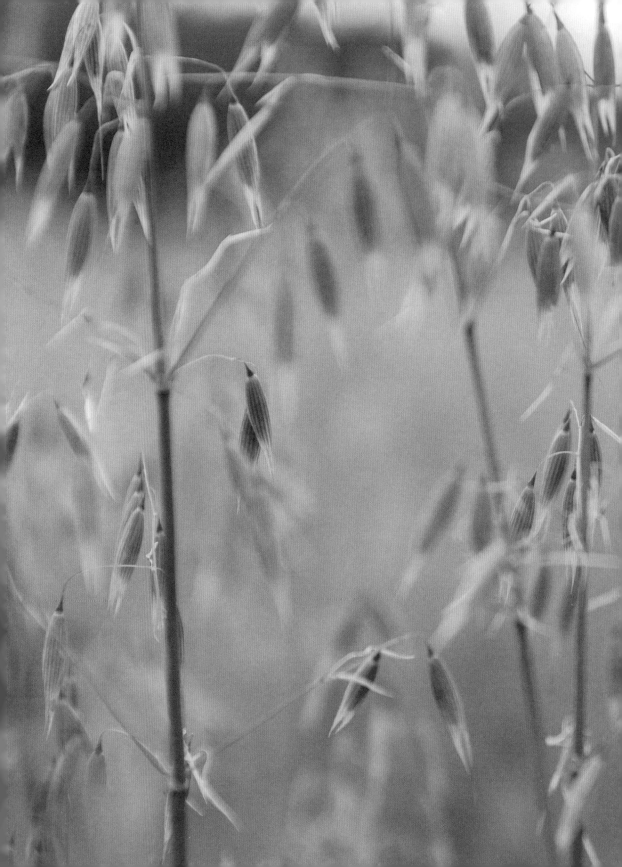

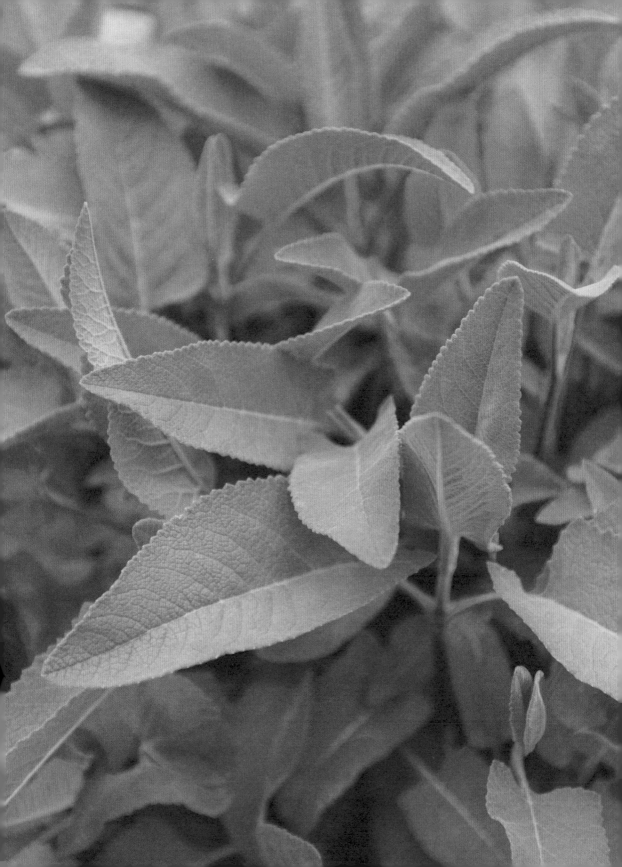

OIL INFUSIONS

Oil infusions are a totally approachable way to extract the therapeutic elements of plant medicines.

User-friendly, flexible and foolproof to make, oil infusions are the foundation for balms, creams, salves, massage oils, natural beauty products and much more. Aromatic herbals with strong, natural volatile oil components are a perfect match for oil infusions – think lavender, and the stellar calendula, which is the base of many medicinal skin recipes. Infused oils also make a wonderful addition to the kitchen and are an easy way to add flavour and supercharge your meals. Like anything, we could overcomplicate making oil infusions, but in truth, we can reap the same rewards by using two simple and accessible methods: cool infusion and solar infusion. Both will allow you to creatively infuse oils with ease for your home apothecary. Listed below are a few golden rules for oil infusions. Bearing these in mind, tune in and create with the plant medicines – there are endless combinations and possibilities!

Choose a base oil high in omega-9 oleic acid. Olive, almond, apricot kernel and sunflower oils are all perfect.

Ensure the plant material is organic, or at least spray and chemical free.

Use the plant material in its most appropriate form (fresh or dried). Refer to the list on page 68.

Select the method that best suits your requirements and plant material. Both methods require you to practise a little patience, so be sure to plan ahead with your medicine making!

To supercharge the medicinal strength, create a double infusion by straining out your plant material after 2–3 weeks, then add a fresh batch of plant material to infuse for another 2–3 weeks.

Keep away from direct sunlight. Store your ready-to-use oils in a cool, dark area – a cupboard is perfect.

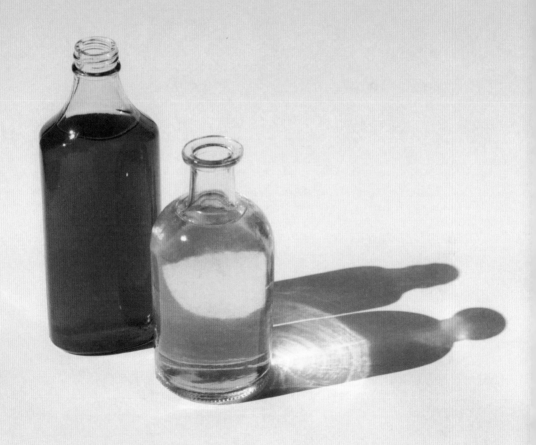

BEST USED DRY

Calendula
Chamomile
Dandelion flowers
Fennel
Garlic
Ginger
Gotu kola
Lavender
Lemon balm
Motherwort
Mugwort
Nettle
Oregano

BEST USED FRESH

Chickweed
Mullein
Passionflower
Peppermint
Red clover
Rosehips
Rosemary
Sage
St John's wort
Thyme
Tulsi
Yarrow

Dried herbs are generally more reliable for producing a beautiful oil infusion (with less risk of excess water creating mould formation), but there are some exceptions to this, where fresh is best. If you are using fresh plant material for your oil infusion, there are a couple of tips to note:

+ Ensure the plants are free of dampness, shake off any soil, and let them sit out and wilt for 12–24 hours before use. This reduces excess moisture in the plant material and allows it to dry out.

+ When your oil infusion is complete, avoid squeezing out the plant material too firmly. This will prevent extra moisture release from the plants.

Use the list above to guide you when creating your infusions.

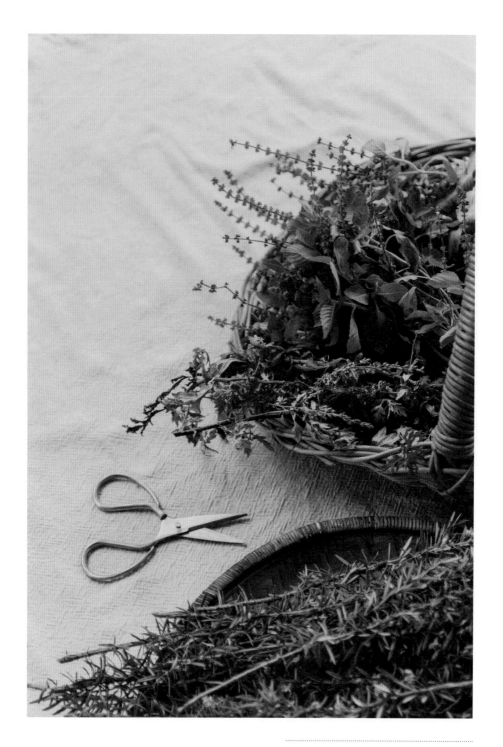

ABOVE: A fragrant trio of garden-grown
and freshly harvested holy basil,
mugwort and rosemary

Cool method oil infusion

This folk recipe is the simplest approach to infusing oils. The easiest road to success here is to use dry plant material – it eradicates the chances of any mishaps with excess moisture and mould formation. I recommend this method for your first oil infusion!

INGREDIENTS

plant material of choice
oil base of choice (e.g.
   olive, almond, apricot
   or sunflower)

EQUIPMENT

scissors
sterilised dry jar and lid
sterilised knife
muslin or fine-mesh sieve

METHOD

Cut the plant material with scissors into coarse pieces.

Fill the sterilised jar with the plant material, leaving around 5–8 cm (2–3 inches) of space at the top. Fully cover the plant material with the chosen oil, then press down and stir with a sterilised knife to release any air pockets – this will create more room in the jar for extra oil.

Top up the jar with an extra 2.5 cm (1 inch) of oil, which should float above the plant material and protect against mould formation. Seal tightly with the sterilised lid and place in a cool, dry, dark environment (a cupboard is perfect).

Visit the oil every few days and give it a gentle shake – not too vigorously, though, as you want to keep the plant material covered by the oil.

Let the oil infuse for 4–6 weeks. The oil will generally take on a deeper colour when it is ready. Once your oil is ready, strain out the plant matter through muslin or with a fine-mesh sieve, and decant your medicinal oil either back into the jar or into a fresh amber glass jar.

Seal and label, noting the date created, type of oil and plant ingredients used. Store in a cool, dry, dark place to preserve longevity and the plant powers.

Solar method oil infusion

Another accessible folk approach to infusing oils. Many herbalists suggest utilising the solar method only for a herb like St John's wort, which needs to be used fresh to activate and extract the medicinal properties. Others feel that the sun is the ultimate way to infuse all oils, with dried or fresh plants. Follow your instincts and see which method works better for you.

INGREDIENTS

plant material of choice
oil base of choice (e.g. olive, almond, apricot or sunflower)

EQUIPMENT

scissors
sterilised dry jar and lid
sterilised knife
muslin or fine-mesh sieve

METHOD

Cut the plant material with scissors into coarse pieces.

Place the plants in the jar, leaving around 5–8 cm (2–3 inches) of space at the top. Fully cover the plant material with the chosen oil, then press down and stir with a sterilised knife to release any air pockets – this will create more room in the jar for extra oil.

Top up the jar with an extra 2.5 cm (1 inch) of oil, which should float above the plant material and protect against mould formation.

Place the sealed jar in a warm, sunny location – a windowsill or lovely garden spot is ideal. Remember to visit the jar every few days and give it a gentle shake.

Let the oil infuse for 4–6 weeks, before straining out the plant matter and decanting.

Seal and label, noting the date created, type of oil and plant ingredients used. Store in a cool, dry, dark place to preserve longevity and the plant powers.

If you are using fresh plant material, such as St John's wort, wilt the harvested plant parts for 24 hours prior to infusing to reduce moisture that may lead to spoilage.

TINCTURES

Tinctures are the most common form of plant medicine that modern clinical herbalists work with and prescribe. Understandably so, as these preparations are shelf-stable and open up a world of possibility for formulations and individualised prescriptions.

Tinctures are single plant extracts, essentially a plant material mixed with alcohol for preservation. Sometimes glycerine is used instead of alcohol to create a glycetract extract (essentially a tincture, yet technically called an extract as it lacks alcohol). This method is suitable for certain herbs, such as marshmallow, and wonderful if you would like to avoid alcohol entirely. In truth, though, the alcohol in your daily dose of a herbal tincture is minuscule! Alcohol is a wonderful solvent, as it holds the medicinal components of the plant and delivers them into the body with ease.

It may take a little trial and error to find your flow with tincture making, but you are guaranteed a rewarding bounty when your plant medicines are ready for use. There are many complex methods for making tinctures, but let's keep it simple and follow the easy folk method.

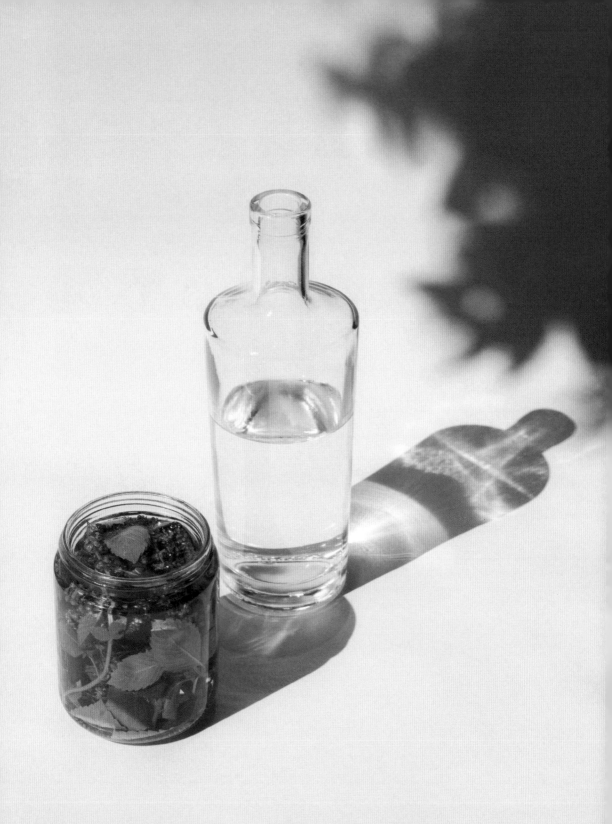

Folk method tincture

A simple, no-fuss approach to tincture making, requiring little equipment and time.

INGREDIENTS
plant material, dried
  or fresh
80–100 proof alcohol –
  vodka is ideal, with its
  neutral flavour

EQUIPMENT
scissors or knife
sterilised dry jar with
  a plastic lid
sheesecloth
stainless steel, wide-
  mouthed funnel
1 litre (34 fl oz/4 cups)
  sterilised amber glass
  bottle with lid

METHOD
Begin by chopping the plant material and adding it to the sterilised jar. If you are using dried bark, berries or roots, ensure they are very finely chopped. The amount you put into the jar will depend on the type of plant material you are using – see note on ratios opposite.

Pour the vodka (otherwise known as the menstruum) over the plant material, covering the herbs well and filling the jar to the brim. To avoid any mould formation, the herbs must be covered at all times with the menstruum.

Seal the jar tightly with the plastic lid (metal lids are susceptible to erosion, so if you must use a metal lid, add a layer of baking paper between the lid and the menstruum, then seal tightly).

Store in a dry, cool place, and visit the tincture every few days to give it a shake and some good vibes! Ensure all of the plant material is covered with the menstruum; double-check after you give it a little shake. Top it up with extra alcohol if need be and reseal. Tinctures prefer taking their time to brew, so practise patience and allow 4–8 weeks.

Once the tincture is ready, it is time to strain out the herbs. Take your cheesecloth and wet it slightly, then lay it over the mouth of the stainless steel funnel. Let the funnel sit in the neck of your sterilised amber glass bottle. Pour the tincture into the cheesecloth, allowing the liquid to drain into the bottle; help it along by squeezing out the plant material vigorously. When drained, compost your plant material.

Seal with the lid, and label the bottle with date made, solvent used and plant ingredients. Store in a cool, dry, low-light area, like a cupboard. The good news is that tinctures basically last forever!

This is a potent plant medicine, so it is best to dose only as needed and aim for 5 ml (1 teaspoon) to a maximum of 15 ml (3 teaspoons) daily in divided doses (e.g. 5 ml three times daily). Dosing more frequently is helpful if you are experiencing acute symptoms.

PLANT MATERIAL RATIOS

The amount of plant material needed for the tincture
recipe will vary depending on the form.

Dried leaves and flowers
Fill around half of the jar with plant material

Fresh leaves and flowers
Fill around three quarters of the jar with plant material

Dried roots, berries, bark
Fill around a quarter of the jar with plant material

Fresh roots, berries, bark
Fill around half of the jar with plant material

OXYMELS AND VINEGARS

Oxymels and vinegars are ancient forms of medicine that have been utilised over the ages, and for good reason. These plant medicines store well and are incredibly easy to make and take daily.

An oxymel is a simple blend of herbs, vinegar and honey. Oxymels harmoniously blend sour and sweet, softening the sharper edges for the tastebuds. They make raw garlic easier to ingest for a cold and flu, which is quite a feat.

A vinegar is very lo-fi way to prepare plant medicines with one base ingredient – vinegar! A wonderful way to infuse fresh or dried herbs, vinegars work beautifully and are incredibly simple to make. They are truly lovely on your salad as a dressing or diluted in warm water as a daily tonic. You can even use herbal vinegars as cleansing hair rinses.

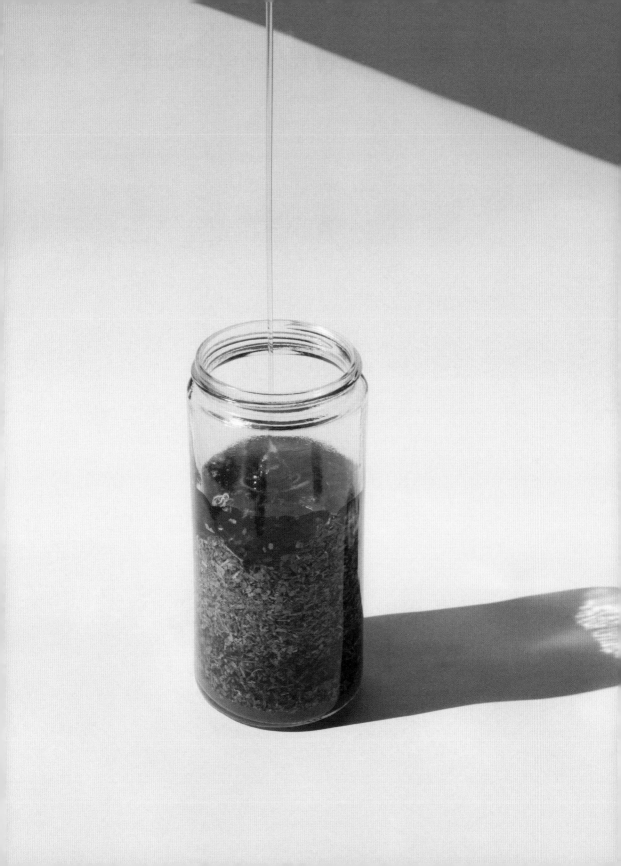

'Tune in' intuition-enhancing oxymel

A recipe gifted by my herbalist soul-sister Lauren Haynes of Wooden Spoon Herbs, from the Appalachian Mountains of Georgia. Lauren's plant medicines are legendary, and, lucky for us all, this blend contains her magical insight. This oxymel combines aromatic plants with a simple folksy approach to medicine making, yielding a divine treat that will strengthen your psychic antennae. You can take it neat, or add to sparkling water for a luscious, refreshing beverage.

INGREDIENTS
1 cup dried tulsi leaf
1 cup dried mugwort
   leaf/flowers
½ cup dried lavender
   flowers
unpasteurised raw apple
   cider vinegar
raw local honey

EQUIPMENT
1 litre (34 fl oz/4 cups)
   sterilised dry jar and lid
baking paper

METHOD
Combine your dried herbal ingredients in the sterilised jar. Pour over the vinegar until the jar looks half full.

Top off the remaining space with raw honey.

Place a piece of baking paper over the top of your preparation, then secure with the lid. Label with the plant ingredients used, date made and any other pertinent information.

Place your jar in front of a sunny window to infuse, shaking it daily. Let it sit for half a moon cycle, or around 2 weeks, before you strain and enjoy.

OXYMEL COMBINATIONS
These are a few delicious suggestions to try, using the method above, but truthfully the possibilities are endless.

Elderberry, mullein, red clover, tulsi
To support and boost immunity and combat a cold or flu.

Red clover, raspberry leaf, nettle leaf
A mineral-rich tonic combination to enhance nourishment and replenish.

Turmeric, ginger, lemon balm
To release the sunshine, lifting the mind, body and spirit.

Gotu kola, tulsi, oat straw, rosemary
To activate and enhance the power of the brain.

The simplest herbal vinegar

I strongly suggest using an unpasteurised raw apple cider vinegar as the base for this recipe. Apple cider vinegar is naturally fermented and has a long list of health benefits; coupling it with fresh herbs is beneficial for gut health and a zingy experience for the palate.

INGREDIENTS

fresh herbs, chopped
unpasteurised raw apple
   cider vinegar

EQUIPMENT

1 litre (34 fl oz/4 cups)
   sterilised dry jar
   and lid
fine-mesh sieve
1 litre (34 fl oz/4 cups)
   sterilised bottle
   with lid

METHOD

Pack the jar around three quarters full with fresh herbs. If using dried herbs, reduce the amount to fill around a quarter of the jar. Pour the apple cider vinegar over the herbs and fill to the top of the jar. Secure the lid tightly. Give the mix a good shake, and pop into a cool, dry, dark cupboard for 2–6 weeks.

The vinegar should have a herb-dense smell and an earthy pungency to it when it is ready for use.

Shake to awaken the vinegar, and strain out the herbs. Decant into the sterilised bottle, ready for use. Best kept in the fridge.

VINEGAR COMBINATIONS

We are spoilt for choice when it comes to making vinegars, with so many combinations and medicinal blends possible. Here are a few favourites.

Dandelion leaves, nettle leaves, gotu kola leaves
This wild-weed green blend amps up nutrition and nourishment, and is best made with fresh plant material.

Nasturtium flowers, nasturtium leaves, rosemary sprigs
A beautiful, peppery, uplifting blend. It is essential to use freshly picked nasturtium in this mix.

Turmeric, garlic cloves, sliced onion, ginger, rosemary sprigs, oregano sprigs, thyme sprigs, sliced lemon, optional fresh chillies, raw honey
A take on a traditional fire cider tonic, seriously immune stimulating and not for the faint-hearted! This mix is best made with fresh ingredients, many of which can be garden grown and are easy to access.

Cinnamon stick, yarrow leaf, rose petals
A light, refreshing vinegar with a gentle floral note, best made with dried plant material.

SYRUPS AND ELIXIRS

Syrups and elixirs are by far the most delicious way to take your plant medicines, adding sweetness and charm.

These delightful preparations detour around the need for a strong preservative or solvent, such as alcohol, and are very agreeable to ingest. Kids love herbal syrups and elixirs, which will feel like a big win for any parent offering medicinal plant remedies!

The difference between syrups and elixirs is the consistency – a syrup is generally thicker than an elixir. Both are nutritious condensed extracts of comforting plant magic.

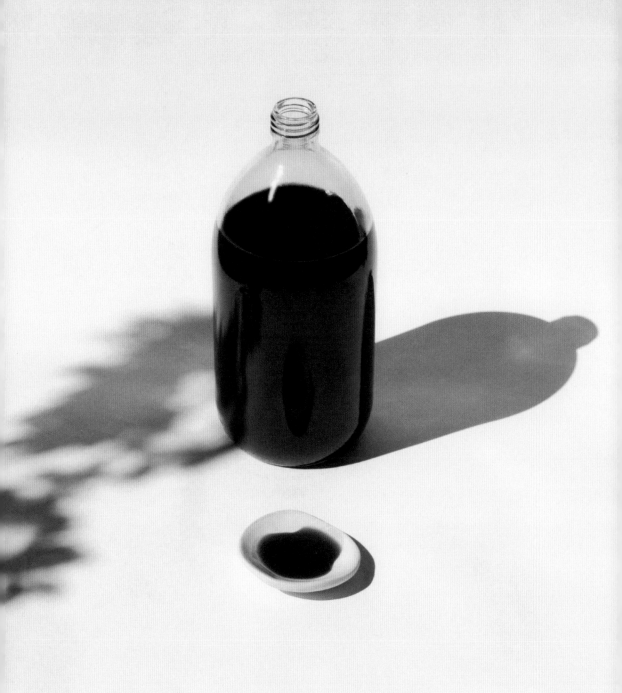

Foundational herbal syrup

This recipe yields a delicious syrup and creates a guideline for infinite herbal possibilities. As long as you follow the quantity of ingredients suggested, fresh or dried, you can make all sorts of wonderful combinations with any herbal-infusion base. The wonderfully wise naturopath Sarah Mann has shared this much-loved recipe, from her green herbal heart to yours.

INGREDIENTS

4 cups spring or filtered water (avoid tap water)
1 cup dried herbs, or 2 cups fresh herbs
1 cup sweetener (raw honey, manuka honey or brown rice syrup)

EQUIPMENT

fine-mesh sieve
saucepan
500 ml (17 fl oz/2 cups) sterilised dry bottle and lid

METHOD

Prepare the herbal infusion with filtered or spring water and allow to infuse to the desired strength.

Strain the herbs through the sieve and pour the infusion into the saucepan. Simmer the liquid on a low heat until it is reduced by approximately half. Remove from heat.

When the reduced infusion has cooled a little but is still warm, add your sweetener of choice and stir until dissolved. (To retain the medicinal enzymes in honey, avoid 'cooking' it – hence keeping the mix at a warm temperature, just enough to allow the sweetener to dissolve with ease.)

Pour the syrup into the sterilised bottle, label clearly with ingredients and the date made, allow it to cool and then store in the fridge for up to 2 months.

SYRUP COMBINATIONS

As wonderful as the following combinations are, please do not underestimate how perfect syrups are with just a single ingredient, such as chamomile, passionflower, cinnamon, rosehip or peppermint.

Rosehip, turmeric, ginger
The perfect winter trio for immune support.

Yarrow, elder leaf, peppermint
The classic Y.E.P. tea combination for colds, fevers and flu.

Licorice, cinnamon, thyme
A combination to stimulate warmth within and build vitality.

Lemon balm, nettle leaf, lavender
A calming and nourishing blend.

Garlic, oregano, orange peel
A strong antimicrobial formula to beat the bugs and enhance immune and gut defences.

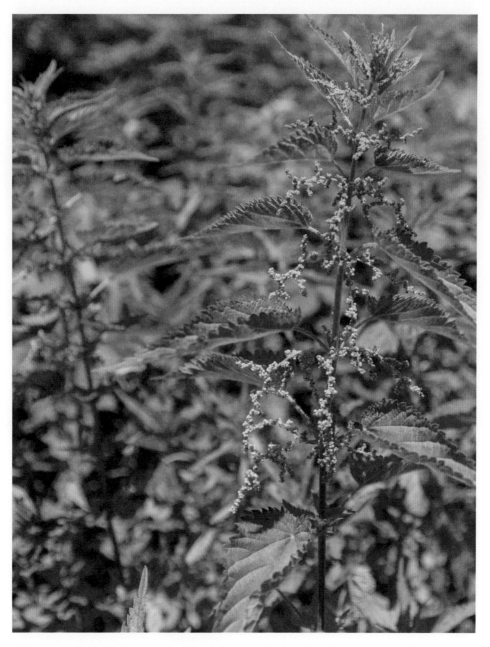

A standard herbal syrup dose is ½ teaspoon–
1 tablespoon, one to three times daily, depending
on your needs. Generally, for deep immune support
while unwell, head towards the higher dose;
for wellness maintenance, a once-daily dose is
beautiful. You can further preserve the syrup with
2 tablespoons of brandy or 2 drops of high-quality
food-grade lemon essential oil, but this is not a must.

ABOVE: Nettle, nourishing and vital

Elderberry elixir

I called upon the queen of the elderberry elixir herself, my mentor and friend, the talented naturopath Kira Sutherland, to share this winter warmer. Kira has been making this uplifting recipe for years, and I am thrilled to share it with you.

INGREDIENTS

200 g (7 oz) fresh elderberries or
   100 g (3½ oz) dried elderberries
60 g (2 oz) dried rosehips
40 g (1½ oz) echinacea roots/
   leaves/flowers
30 g (1 oz) cinnamon chips
15 g (½ oz) licorice root
2 litres (68 fl oz/8 cups) apple juice
   or 1½ litres (51 fl oz/6 cups) apple
   juice and 500 ml (17 fl oz/2 cups)
   pomegranate juice (be sure to use
   sugar-free fruit juices)
300 ml (10 fl oz/1¼ cups) raw
   honey

EQUIPMENT

large saucepan
fine-mesh sieve
sterilised glass bottles and lids

METHOD

Place all of the herbal ingredients in the saucepan and add the 2 litres (68 fl oz/8 cups) of juice. Mix gently. Bring to the boil over a medium heat, then simmer for 1–1½ hours, stirring occasionally. Remove from the heat and allow to cool.

Strain out the herbs through a fine-mesh sieve. Put the liquid back on the stove and add the raw honey. Stir over very low heat until the honey has melted through (avoid overheating the honey, so as to preserve its enzyme-rich properties).

Allow the mix to cool completely, then decant into sterilised glass bottles or jars. Seal well and store in the fridge for up to a month.

This mix is delicious straight off the spoon!
Take 1 tablespoon daily for wellness, and
increase up to 3 tablespoons daily if immunity
is feeling a little depleted.

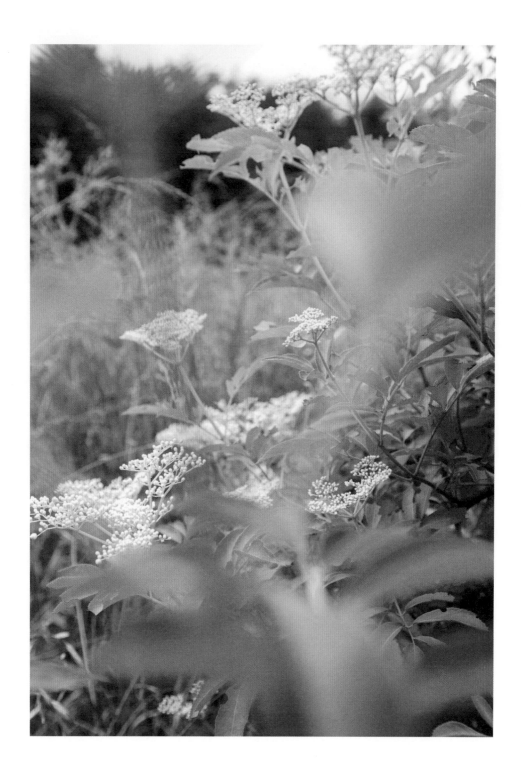

ABOVE: Wild-growing elder in bloom

BALMS AND CREAMS

Modern skincare preparations can be a minefield to navigate. Often the ingredients list is full of near-unrecognisable items. Whipping up your own products is a fun, empowering process, with the assurance of purity of ingredients and plant-powered therapeutics.

The skin is our largest organ; it is our protective barrier, shielding and supporting. Often when the skin needs extra TLC, plant medicine–rich balms and creams have a knack for healing with profound efficacy. The good news is that if you have created a simple oil infusion using one of the methods on pages 70–1, you are well on your way to blending balms and creams like a pro! Herbal oil infusions provide the medicinal base for balms and creams, and there are so many wonderful possibilities.

There is a big difference between a balm and a cream. Creams are water based, making them more prone to spoilage, and therefore they need to be refrigerated. Creams are wonderful for beauty applications and moisturising the skin.

Balms are oil based, making them more stable. They are commonly used in medicinal, healing applications to soothe cuts, scrapes, rashes and bites.

I turned to my friend Justina Edwards of Being Skincare, the master mixologist of all things medicinal for the skin, to share her go-to recipes and approach to making balms and creams.

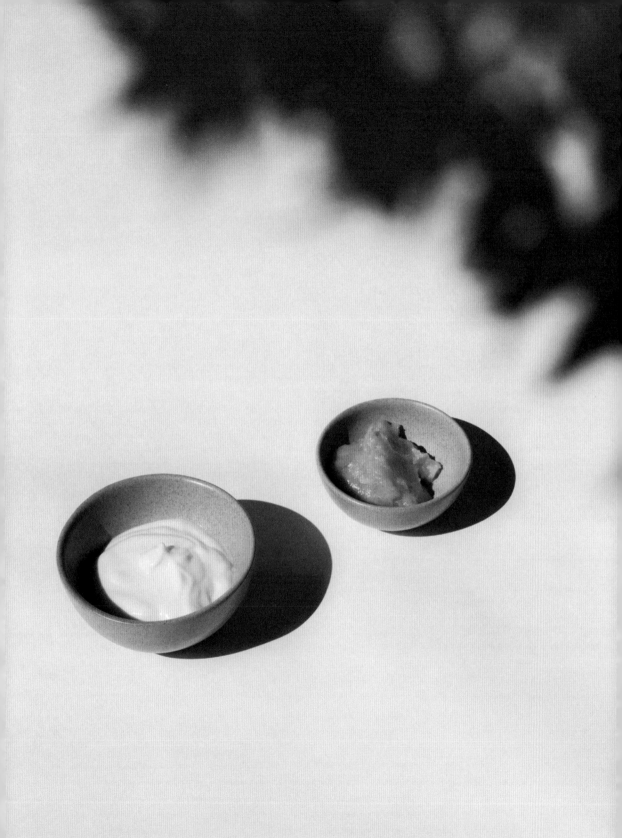

Essential medicinal balm

Use this easy-to-navigate recipe to create the perfect balm and as a golden guide for experimenting with the different combinations suggested below. Makes roughly 1 cup.

INGREDIENTS

200 ml (7 fl oz) infused oil(s) of your choice
40 g (1½ oz) beeswax
vitamin E oil (optional)

EQUIPMENT

double boiler or sterilised glass jar and saucepan
stainless steel teaspoon
5 x 50 ml (1¾ fl oz) sterilised glass jars and lids

METHOD

Put the infused oil(s) and beeswax in a double boiler. If you don't have a double boiler, put the ingredients in a sterilised glass jar, then sit the jar in a saucepan with 2.5 cm (1 inch) of water in the bottom. Stir continuously over low heat until the beeswax has fully melted and combined with the oil.

Dip a stainless steel teaspoon into the mixture, then place in the fridge on a sheet of baking paper for 5 minutes to test the viscosity. If you are seeking a more solid balm, add a little extra beeswax to firm it up; if you desire a softer balm, simply add a dash more oil and test again until the desired consistency is achieved.

Remove from the heat and add a couple of drops of vitamin E oil to slow oxidation and extend shelf life, if desired. Pour the mixture into the sterilised glass jars.

Place paper towel over the tops of the jars and allow to cool completely – overnight is best. This prevents the balm from 'sinking' in the middle.

In the morning, pop on the lids and labels. Remember to include the ingredients, instructions for use and use-by date. This formula should last for one year.

BALM COMBINATIONS

Healing balm

Create an infusion of lavender, gotu kola, chickweed and calendula flowers in olive oil, then make a balm using the above formula. This is a nice all-purpose blend, and what I love about these herbs is that they are easy to wildcraft or grow in your backyard.

Menstrual cramp balm

Create an infusion of lavender, chamomile flowers and peppermint leaf in olive oil. To make the balm, mix 150 ml (5 fl oz) of the infused oil with 50 ml (1¾ fl oz) castor oil, then follow the go-to medicinal balm formula as above. Add a quarter of a teaspoon of cayenne pepper to the oil–wax emulsion at the end and stir in gently.

The lovely cream formula

Justina's perfectly balanced recipe is based on the grandmother of herbal medicine Rosemary Gladstar's beloved Perfect Cream. It allows you to get as creative as you want, as long as you stick to the measurements below – so you can divide the base oil measurement into parts if using a combination of oils, for example. You can experiment with different hydrosols (aromatic water or steam distillations of plant material), or even herbal infusions. If using herbal tea or water-based infusions, it's important to note this will drastically reduce the shelf life and the cream will need to be stored in the fridge. Makes roughly 1 cup.

INGREDIENTS
100 ml (3½ fl oz) rosewater or hydrosol of your choosing
50 ml (1¾ fl oz) aloe vera gel
110 ml (3¾ fl oz) base oil, such as olive, almond, apricot or avocado oil
40 ml (1½ fl oz) solid or semi-solid melted oil, such as coconut oil, cocoa butter or shea butter
15 g (½ oz) beeswax
vitamin E oil (optional)

EQUIPMENT
small bowl
double boiler or sterilised glass jar and saucepan
500 ml (17 fl oz/2 cups) sterilised glass jar
stick (immersion) blender with whisk attachment
wooden skewer or clean chopstick
6 x 50 ml (1¾ fl oz) sterilised glass jars and lids

METHOD

Combine the rosewater and aloe vera gel in a small bowl and set aside.

Put the oils and beeswax in a double boiler. If you don't have a double boiler, put the ingredients in a sterilised glass jar, then sit the jar in a saucepan with 2.5 cm (1 inch) of water in the bottom. Stir continuously over low heat until the beeswax has fully melted and combined with the oil.

Remove from the heat and add a couple of drops of vitamin E oil to slow oxidation and extend shelf life, if desired. Pour into the sterilised glass jar and allow to cool to room temperature.

Once the oils have cooled, start drizzling in the rosewater and aloe vera mixture while whisking with the stick blender on a slow speed. Be sure to do this slowly so the water-based ingredients can emulsify with the oils. Watch for the mixture to become thick and creamy. Do not overdo it – test at intervals until the desired consistency has been achieved.

Stir with a wooden skewer or clean chopstick at the end to make sure all of the ingredients have been combined, then transfer to the sterilised glass jars and seal.

CREAM COMBINATIONS
After-sun cream
Replace the rosewater with a strong herbal water infusion of peppermint, but bear in mind the cream will have a shorter shelf life, as noted above. Stored in the fridge, this is a heavenly combination. The peppermint counteracts heat with fresh minty coolness while the aloe vera soothes sun-drenched skin.

Nourishing softness cream
Create an oil infusion of calendula flowers and lavender in your oil base of choice. Use this gentle combination for the oil portion of the cream recipe to enhance skin glow and suppleness.

BATHS AND STEAMS

It is often the simplest remedies that give us the most relief and fulfilment. Herbal baths and steams absolutely fit this category. They are both underrated and under-utilised in our everyday lives. They offer an opportunity to unwind and let go, to step outside of the doing space into a more receiving energy. The body loosens and the brain calms, stress begins to untangle, and the breath eases.

Herbal baths are luxurious, yet oh-so-easy to pull together after a long day. A particularly beautiful ritual, herbal foot baths can be prepared and enjoyed with ease and accessibility by all. Steams offer speedy relief for a congested respiratory system, opening up nasal passages and encouraging the lungs to clear.

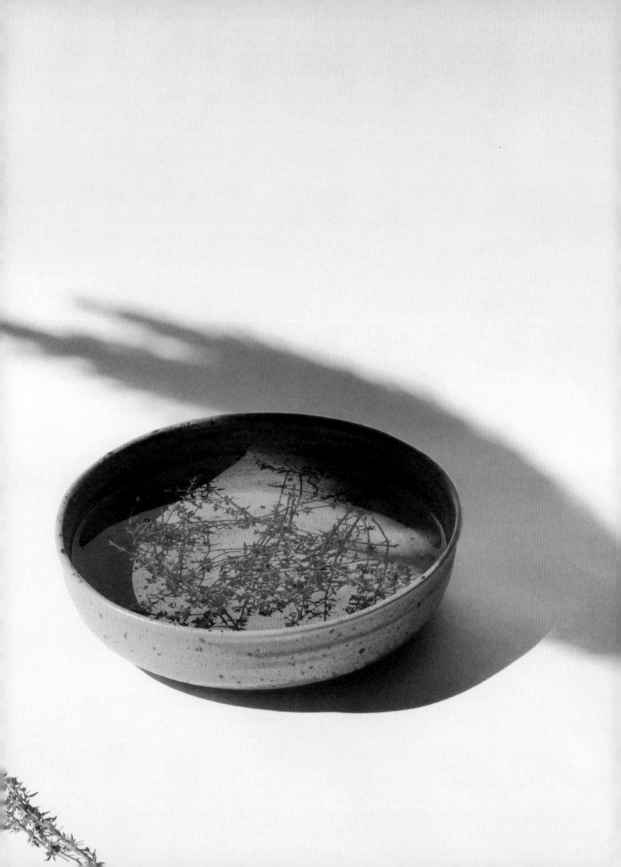

Herbal foot bath

Use aromatic herbs for this wonderfully simple ritual – see the combinations suggested below. You want to ignite the senses and bring all parts of your being into the present moment. This is a powerful act of self-care – enjoy it!

INGREDIENTS

5 tablespoons blended herbs
water

EQUIPMENT

large saucepan with lid
fine-mesh sieve (optional)
basin (large enough to accommodate your feet)
comfy chair
towel

METHOD

Add your herbs to the saucepan and fill with water. Bring to a rapid boil and simmer for 10–15 minutes with the lid on to keep in the volatile aromatic elements of the plants. Remove from the heat and strain out the herbs, if desired, or keep them happily floating around as you pour the mix into the basin.

Add cold water to the mix to ensure the foot bath is comfortable but still as hot as possible.

Position yourself comfortably in your favourite chair, with a towel alongside for drying your feet when you are finished. Gently immerse your feet in the basin – ideally the water will be deep enough to cover your ankles. Relax, breathe, unwind.

Stay here for as long as you feel you need to – at least 10 minutes is ideal.

HERBAL BATH COMBINATIONS

These can all be made with either fresh or dried herbs and used in your bath or foot bath.

Rosemary sprigs, oregano sprigs
An invigorating, protective blend.

Rose petals, lavender
A relaxing, bliss-inducing combination.

Sage, nettle leaf and fresh lemon
A refreshing trio for weary, overworked feet.

Lemon balm, rose petals, chamomile flowers
A sweet and soft blend to decompress the nervous system and refuel the heart.

Simple steam inhalation

Steam inhalations really shine for nasal and lung congestion, particularly when you are under the weather with a cold or flu. The plant medicines that are indicated for steam inhalations, such as those suggested below, are often fragrant and rich in natural volatile oils, perfect for sensory clearing of the body.

INGREDIENTS
1 heaped tablespoon
  fresh or dried herb(s)
boiling water

EQUIPMENT
heatproof bowl
towel

METHOD
Add your herbs to the heatproof bowl, pour boiling water over and stir gently.

To avoid any steam burns, ensure you leave a decent distance between your face and the bowl – please test this first with your hand.

Cloak yourself with a towel and lean over the bowl with your face directly above the steaming brew.

Close your eyes and take deep inhalations through the nose for up to 5 minutes.

When you feel ready, emerge from your steamy cocoon and allow any mucus to come up and out if need be.

STEAM COMBINATIONS
These can all be made with either fresh or dried herbs.

Thyme, fresh lemon
Antibacterial and clearing to the sinus passages; shakes and breaks up phlegm.

Peppermint, rosemary
Stimulating, energising and decongesting.

Sage, mullein
A soothing combination for any bronchial issues, clearing restriction and stagnation.

Plants for the People

JELLIES AND PASTILLES

Making herbal jellies and pastilles is a super-clever way to encourage little ones, and grown-ups in a sensitive state, to take their dose of plant medicine.

Jelly brings many of us a nostalgic reminder of childhood, a treat wired into our subconscious. A trick of the herbal trade, jelly is used to disguise stronger-flavoured tinctures, infusions and powders, while being kind of fun to eat and experience!

Pastilles are a soft lozenge of sorts. They are easy to make and are particularly helpful for red, raw sore throats, angry mouth ulcers and upper respiratory tract congestion and infections. They dissolve with ease in the mouth and are simply made with herbal powders, liquids and honey.

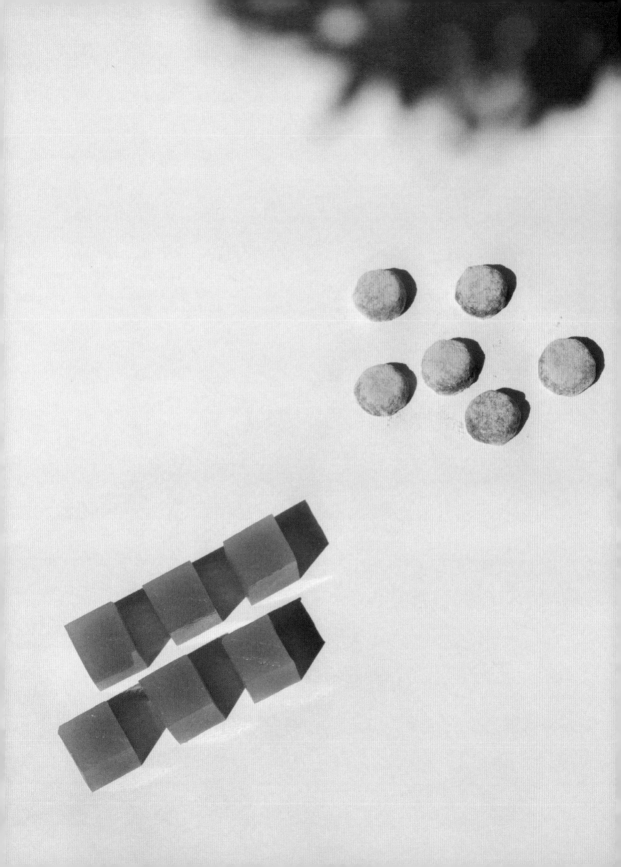

Herbal pastilles

This is a recipe from my dear naturopathic sister Sarah Mann, using slippery elm bark powder as the main binding agent. Slippery elm coats and soothes sore throats and irritated respiratory passages – simply couple with your herbal infusion and powder of choice in this versatile medicinal recipe. Makes 12–15 pastilles.

INGREDIENTS

1–2 tablespoons raw honey, rice malt syrup or manuka honey
¼ cup warm, strong herbal infusion
½ cup slippery elm powder
1 tablespoon dry powdered herb(s)
fine edible powder, to dust (e.g. slippery elm powder, brown rice flour or cinnamon)

EQUIPMENT

bowl
baking paper
rolling pin
dehydrator (optional)

METHOD

In a bowl, stir the raw honey (or your sticky sweetener of choice) into your warm herbal infusion until dissolved. Add the slippery elm powder and powdered dry herbs to the bowl and combine thoroughly to form a thick but not crumbly dough.

Shape the dough into 12–15 small balls and place on a sheet of baking paper. Cover with another sheet of baking paper and roll the balls flat with a rolling pin.

Uncover and lightly dust with the edible powder. Leave to air-dry for a day, or place in a dehydrator on a low setting to dry. Store in an airtight container and use within 6–8 weeks.

PASTILLE COMBINATIONS

Soft and zingy
Lemon balm infusion with cinnamon and ginger powder.

Uplifting and stimulating
Peppermint infusion with ginger powder.

Restorative and enhancing
Licorice infusion with ginger powder.

Nourishing and replenishing
Rosehip infusion with turmeric powder and a dash of black pepper.

Soothing and settling
Rose and licorice infusion with ground rose petals and calendula flowers.

Protective and fortifying
Sage and elderberry infusion with cinnamon and ginger powder.

....

Fruit jellies

Although these simple jellies are a hit with kids, they are also a regular feature in many of my adult clients' fridges. You can adjust the fruit–juice ratio and reduce the sugars by adding water instead of juice and increasing the amount of fruit. This is a flexible recipe, easy to make and foolproof. When you are considering the taste of the jelly, try using different fruity flavour combinations to round out the strength of the herbals. Makes two standard ice-cube trays (32 cubes).

INGREDIENTS

5 tablespoons gelatine powder* (or agar-agar powder/flakes for a vegetarian jelly)

1 cup water

1 cup fresh or frozen fruit (organic berries are perfect)

1 cup fruit juice (choose stronger-flavoured juices, such as grape, prune or pear, with no added sugar)

herbal medicine – tincture, infusion, etc. (see dosage information in method)

EQUIPMENT

bowl
saucepan
strainer (optional)
ice-cube trays or moulds

METHOD

Place the gelatine powder and water in a bowl, mix gently and allow the gelatine to 'bloom', absorbing the water for a few minutes.

Place the fruit in a saucepan and mash down a little with a fork over low to medium heat. (If using frozen fruit, allow it to thaw in the heat of the pan first.) Add the fruit juice and stir through until well combined, then add the bloomed gelatine.

Heat until the gelatine becomes liquid, stirring constantly until smooth. At this point you could add a touch of optional sweetener, such as maple syrup.

Remove from the heat and either strain out the fruit for a smooth jelly or keep as is. Pour the liquid into ice-cube trays or moulds (fun shapes gain extra points!) and include a half to full herbal dose as prescribed per cube. For example, if a child needs 2 ml (scant ½ teaspoon) of a strong echinacea infusion, add 2 ml to one mould or divide between two moulds, and then offer the child their daily dose of one or two jellies.

Mix gently and refrigerate to set.

*Ensure gelatine is derived from pasture-raised/grass-fed livestock sources.

If you prefer a softer jelly, simply add an extra half a cup of fruit juice or water.

Gelatine and agar-agar, a seaweed-derived gelatinous thickener, are easy to find at your local health food store.

POULTICES AND WASHES

These are two quick methods for applying plant medicine. Remember them when you are seeking a remedy stat!

Poultices are a method of applying herbs directly to the skin. Made from fresh or dried plants, they are wonderful for burns, splinters, cuts, bites, bruises, skin irritations and infections, menstrual cramps, aches and pains. Poultices require the plant material to be made into a pulp or a paste-like consistency – think grated or powdered ginger with a little hot water. The paste can be made from a single plant or a combination, and a base such as slippery elm powder can be used to create a thicker consistency.

The poultice can be applied directly to the skin in a thick layer, then covered with a soft cotton cloth, or it can be spread between two layers of soft cotton cloth and then applied to the skin. The method of application depends on the type of herb you are using. With ginger, for example, you would choose the latter method to reduce any burning sensation from the fiery paste (unless you desired the heat-inducing direct action). Once the compress has been applied, cover with a towel to contain the effect. You can add a hot water bottle on top for extra warmth, or an ice pack to increase cooling action.

Fresh chickweed, calendula flowers, chamomile flowers and dandelion leaves are perfect for poultices. However, there are many herbs that have an affinity for topical skin support. Even the humble grated potato holds medicinal powers as a poultice, drawing out infections.

Washes are water-based infusions of herbs, best applied locally to a small region of the body. They are wonderful for issues of the eyes, such as conjunctivitis and styes, or for skin infections on the face, such as staph or bacterial acne.

Making a wash is super simple: brew your infusion, then cool and pour a small amount into a clean bowl. Immerse a cotton pad in the wash and soak through. Apply this directly to the affected area. To avoid contamination of the wash, be sure not to double-dip your pad; always use a clean cotton pad for every wash cycle.

Washes can be made from any herbal blend, but the greatest multi-use plant medicine for all skin infection concerns is calendula. Calendula flowers are superbly antiseptic and antiviral, and encourage wound healing.

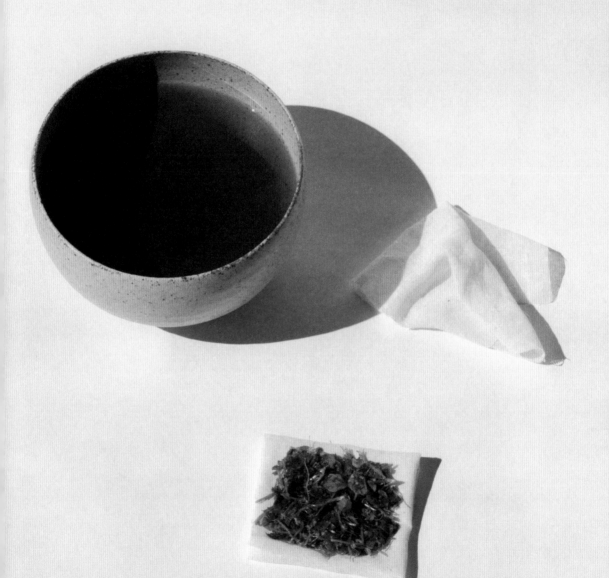

FLOWER ESSENCES

These energetic remedies are divine allies. Purely vibrational in nature, they work on the spiritual and emotional planes via energetic medicine. Dr Edward Bach, the father of flower essences, was ahead of his time when he created Bach flower remedies in the 1930s.

The premise is that flowers hold wisdom, messages, a healing spirit and forces. Once infused in pure spring water and bathed in sunshine, they transmit their vibrational imprint and therapeutic offerings to the remedy. These essences act as deep catalysts for mental, emotional and spiritual transformation and change, working with challenging mind states, stuck emotional patterns and spiritual imbalances. They are so gentle in nature that they are perfectly safe for young ones, elders and all in between. Flower essences have the ability to speak directly to our nervous system, soothing stress and anxiety, lifting moods and mind states, and softening the layers of trauma. After all, we are energetic beings, attuned to the vibrations around us.

Flower essences can be made with ease, but there are some very important practical and esoteric elements to consider as you step into this realm of creation.

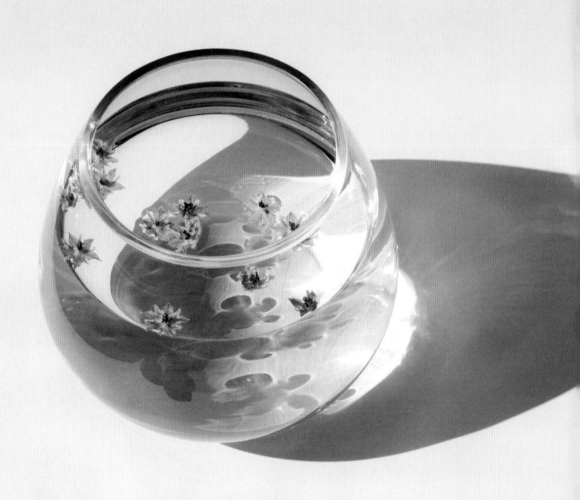

Identifying flowers that are safe to infuse in water is paramount. Do your research to be sure the flower is non-toxic and safe for consumption.

Connect with a flowering plant that calls you; one that you admire frequently or spend time with is a great start. Remember to practise the wildcrafting golden rules on page 35.

Begin with a clear heart, mind and spirit. A little meditation or deep breathing may help to anchor your intentions and bring you into present-time consciousness.

Connect with the plant. It is most important to practise presence during the process of making your essence. This transforms the remedy from a simple flower water to an *essence*; it is all about your deeper connection to the spirit of the plant and accessing your intuition to hear the messages, which form the therapeutic elements of your essence.

Prepare your essence-making tools on a vibrant, sunny day. You will need a clean glass bowl, 100 ml (3½ fl oz) spring water, a clean funnel, a 200 ml (7 fl oz) sterilised amber glass medicine bottle and lid, and 100 ml (3½ fl oz) good-quality brandy to preserve the vibration of the essence in the final stages.

Gently harvest the flowers, being sure not to touch or spoil the blooms. Try to hold onto the leaves where possible.

Fill the bowl with spring water (bottled water is also acceptable) and place the flowers in the bowl to float; aim to cover as much of the surface as possible, allowing them to imbue their essence.

Position the bowl in full sunshine to infuse for up to 4 hours. Essentially this is a water infusion prepared with the aid of the solar forces.

Remember this is basically magic-making, so add any elements or practices that enhance your personal connection to all things magical. You can perhaps surround the bowl with crystals, prayer and intention. Be mindful that any ritual holds a vibration, so all this will infuse your essence too!

The essence is ready to be decanted into your amber glass bottle after infusing. Remove the flowers gently – try to do this with a leaf, twig or plant material where possible. There should be no physical part of the plant present in the final preparation. Pour the infused water into the glass bottle through the funnel. The bottle should be around half full. Fill to the top with the brandy and seal with the lid.

You have created a mother essence! Label with the name of the flower, location made and date, and note the ratio of water to brandy.

Keep your essence in a cool, low-light cupboard. The longevity of a mother flower essence is generally up to ten years.

The mother essence can be used to create many more essences, like essence babies! These are called stock essences. To make a stock essence, create a solution of equal parts spring water and brandy in a sterilised 50 ml (1¾ fl oz) bottle and add 2-3 drops of the mother essence; gently shake to activate. Now you are ready to create a dosage bottle, the most common form of essences you will see on the shelves of health food stores: fill a sterilised 25 ml (¾ fl oz) bottle with a base of three quarters spring water to one quarter brandy, adding 3 drops from the stock bottle. The daily dosage is generally 3 drops under the tongue up to three times throughout the day. Essences are simply gentle-natured; notice how you respond and adjust your dosages accordingly.

Endless possibilities exist with flower-essence remedies. They are a way to tap into the pulse of subtle energies, and remind us that there are depths in nature to be felt far beyond what we may consciously comprehend. Welcome them in.

CEREMONIAL STICKS

Burning plants for healing began with Indigenous peoples. Many cultures and religions worldwide revere sacred plant powers of purification, weaving them into ritual, ceremony and blessings.

Every plant has a spirit, an essence that interacts with unseen forces. The smoke represents a clearing and cleansing ally for the body, mind and spirit, repelling dense energies to make way for clear, fresh energies. With this in mind, these are traditional practices and I urge you to treat them with sincere respect. Our actions and intentions create an impact; as we practise elements of traditional medicine in connection to the earth and the unseen forces, we honour those who have come before us and those who will follow us. Entering into this ceremonial practice with mindfulness and attuned awareness only potentiates the energy and effect.

Creating ceremonial sticks is a beautiful way to use wildcrafted or homegrown fresh plant material in a tactile, creative exercise that can be quite meditative. They are wonderful for cleansing a space and clearing stagnant emotions, setting intentions, celebrations and initiations, aiding sleep and enhancing spiritual insights, grounding the body and lifting mood.

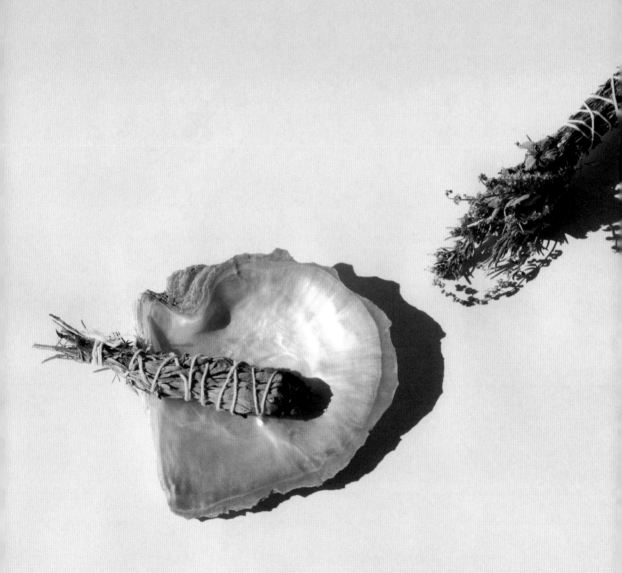

CREATING

Choose aromatic plants rich in volatile oils and scent, such as lavender, garden sage, lemon balm, rosemary, mugwort, tulsi, rose petals, mullein, yarrow, peppermint.

This is an intuitive practice. These are merely guidelines; the practice is open to interpretation and there are no right or wrong combinations!

Prepare your fresh plant material by trimming the length of the stems to around 20–25 centimetres (8–10 inches).

Begin to bundle your plants together in layers. If you have flowering plants, it is extra special to use them as the outer layer so the blooms and buds are visible.

Choose a natural fibre–rich twine or string, such as cotton or hemp, and tie off the plant-bundle base with a sturdy knot, leaving plenty of string on one side to wrap upwards, and enough string on the other side to secure the ends when you have finished wrapping the bundle. Be sure to also leave a little stem at the base to hold when burning your stick.

Draw the plant material together and, holding the bundle in one hand, begin to bind from the base with the excess string, winding upwards at a slight angle with your other hand. This makes it easy to cross the string over at the top and make your way back down to secure any plant material that may be loose or poking out.

Tie off with the leftover length of string at the base of the original knot to secure your stick.

Hang to dry, or store in a dry, low-light area for 3–4 weeks.

IN CEREMONY

Choose a bowl or special vessel to act as a fireproof dish.

Set your intentions and anchor your body, mind and spirit in the present moment.

Holding the base of the bundle in your hand, light the top, allowing the dried plants to catch and create a steady flame. Blow out gently, making way for the smoke stream from the smouldering plants.

Connect with the moment and allow the aromatic plants to awaken your senses.

Move the smoke by fanning it with your spare hand or a feather, allowing the vapours to permeate the space, object, person or intention receiving the ceremony.

When completed, thank the plant spirits and rest the bundle in the fireproof dish to allow the smoke to settle. A quick way to extinguish any burning embers is to submerge the tip of the stick in a little water; this will dry quickly and your ceremonial stick can be called upon again and again.

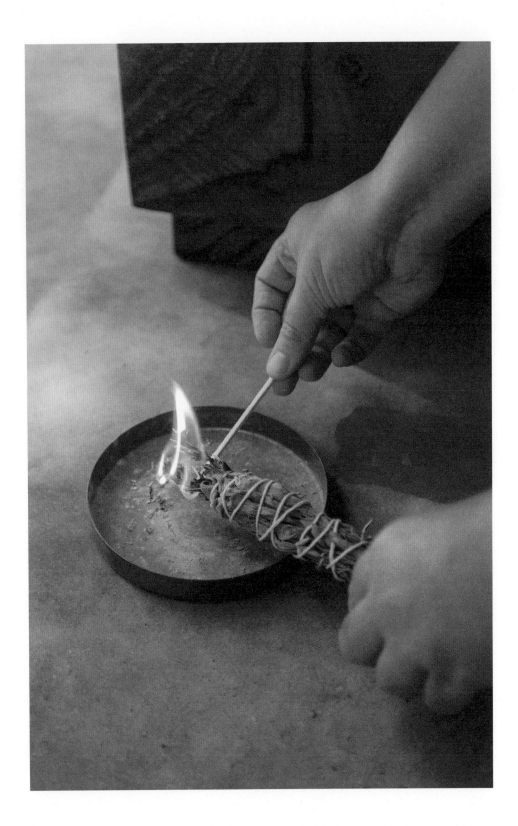

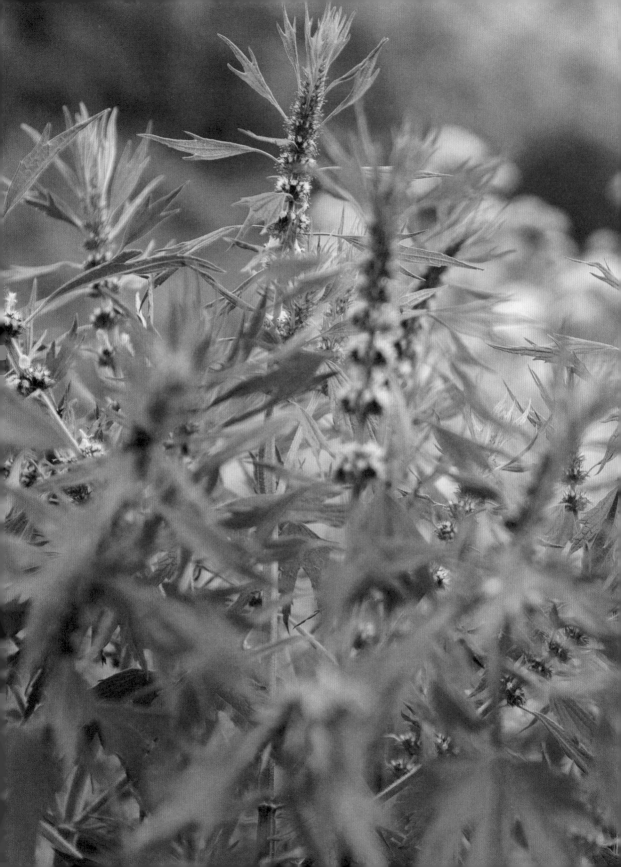

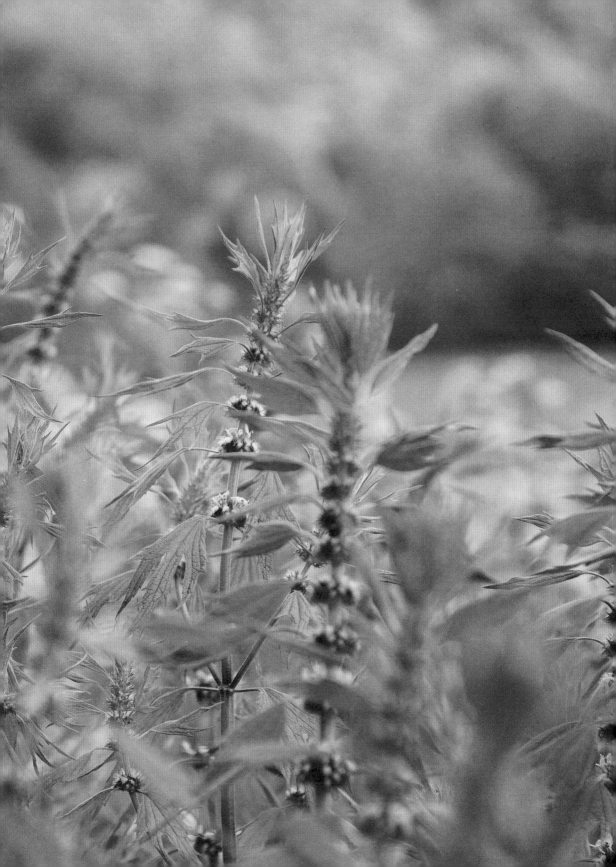

Materia Medica

Materia Medica

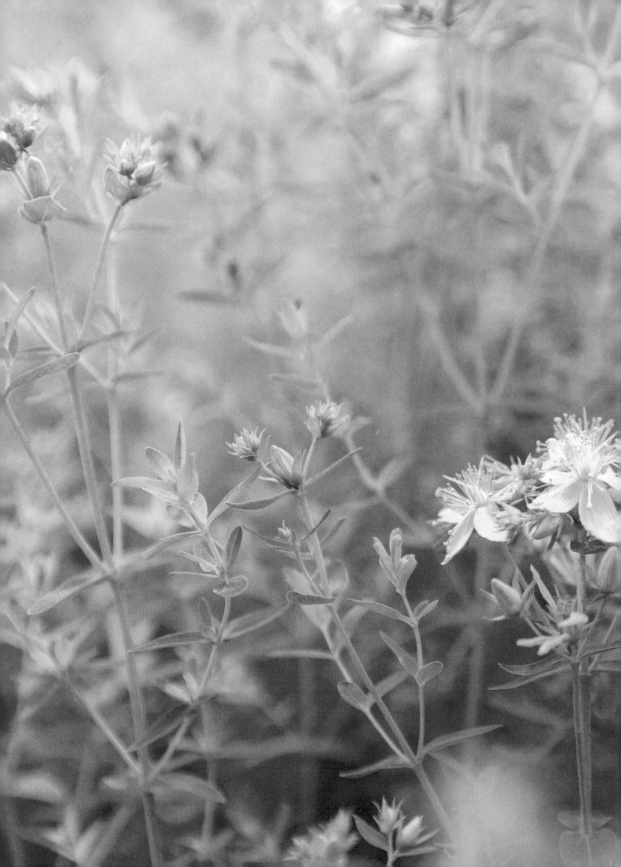

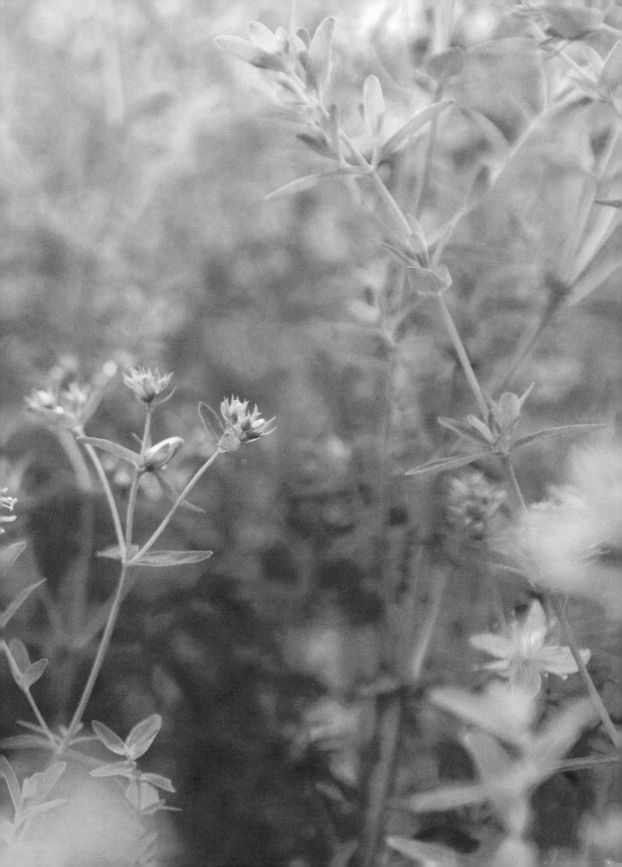

WHOLE PLANT MEDICINE

Every plant has a personality, a story, characteristics, quirks, strengths. There is an undeniable innate synergy that happens when plants and people align.

The term 'whole plant medicine' may be a little misleading to some. It does not mean that the entirety of a plant is used in every herbal preparation; rather, it refers to a wholeness in the approach. Whole plant parts are always used – leaves, roots, barks, berries and flowering heads – as opposed to isolated phytochemical constituents. Nothing has been reduced or pulled apart.

With so much emphasis currently on the biochemical qualities of herbs, I worry we are losing our way, our understanding of the dynamism in whole plant medicine. That we are simplifying yet overcomplicating it all. Our ancestors did not comprehend what an active constituent or isolated compound was; they understood the forces of the whole plant. When we remove one constituent from a plant, do we remove the synergy of the other essential elements that allow the plant to be the full healing force it is?

I would expect the isolated constituent to be effective for certain ailments and presentations. After all, it is still plant medicine, in another form. But the efficacy of whole plant medicine, with its full-bodied vigour, can never be surpassed.

Western herbalism, Chinese medicine, Ayurveda, Greek medicine, folk medicine, Indigenous medicines – these cultures have imparted knowledge and continue to shape our understanding of the powers of plant-based healing. Each methodology has a belief that the energetic properties of a plant must be understood to truly catalyse healing. In other words, we must consider not only the physiological impacts of a plant's healing ability but also the unseen forces. Chinese medicine is rooted in energetic language and meaning. Qi (the life force), Shen (spiritual energy), Jing (the giver of life), Yin (the feminine, inward, cool energy) and Yang (the masculine, outward, warm energy) are all interconnected terms that acknowledge the intangible in the tangible. Ayurveda has the dosha system to define energies in the body and being: Vata, Pitta and Kapha. Other systems look at tissue states, the subtle anatomies (chakras and meridians) and the overall constitution to diagnose and correct energetic imbalances.

There is a vital force within plants and within people. The term 'energetics' is often used to explain the essence of a plant and the forces that lie within it. Energetics can be applied not only to plants but also to ourselves: we are a part of the vibrational footprint. All living things have an electromagnetic field and energetic frequency, and understanding this really amplifies the potential of plant medicine. Finding the best-aligned plant to work with often comes down to the energetics and not just the named physical medicinal actions of a plant. Dis-ease is an indication that the vital force is out of whack, so harmonising support with the vital force is needed. Bring on the plant medicines!

I will add that it is so important to cultivate a connection with your remedy. Enjoy it – grow it if you are able, get to know it. The plants can be cultivated in all sorts of gardens; many can be found growing locally or sourced dried in the aisles of your favourite health food store.

All of the content that lies ahead focuses on emphasising and honouring whole plant use and the therapy plant medicine can offer.

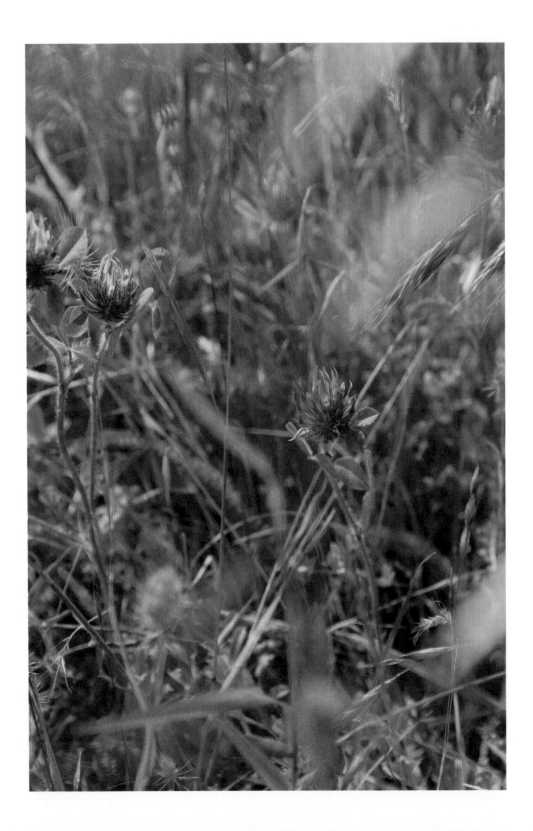

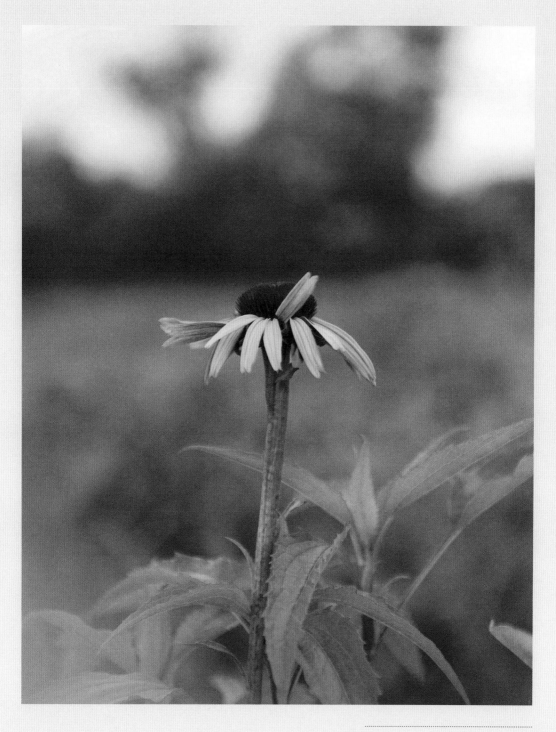

ABOVE: An echinacea flower signals
summer is on the way

LEFT: Red clover, growing wild and free

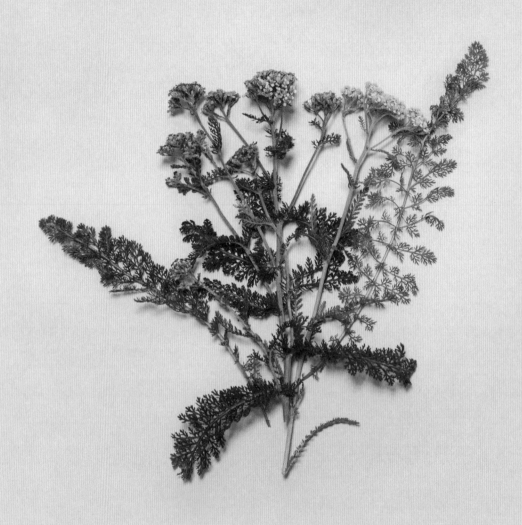

GOLDEN TIP

Yarrow is the perfect herb
for use in a sitz bath during
and post birth to ease excess
blood flow and heal tissues.

ACHILLEA MILLEFOLIUM
YARROW

Associated with the mystical forces, yarrow is deeply embedded in Western herbal medicine. Widespread in Europe and North America, this captivatingly pretty plant has feathery, deep-green leaves and flowering crowns in tones of white and pink. It is also a tough, truly adaptive, commanding plant, willing to protect and meet you where you need to be met. Containing an inherent wisdom recognised by our ancestors, yarrow has been of great service to many ancient cultures and has offered its assistance in times of war, healing the wounds and easing the pains of the brave. Traditional Native American use speaks more to digestive complaints, and to this day we value yarrow for its ability to stimulate an appetite and calm the belly.

Yarrow is the master of the blood, with the capacity to coagulate and cease blood flow, moderating wounds and bruising. From mild uterine or gastrointestinal bleeding to postpartum care and haemorrhoids, yarrow can help to harmonise blood flow. This herbal healer also eases digestive and menstrual cramping, bringing relief. One of yarrow's stellar applications is addressing a fever via its diaphoretic action: by encouraging circulation, it causes sweat to move to the skin's surface, cooling the body and helping to break a fever, while the immune system amplifies defences. Colds and flus respond beautifully to yarrow's medicine. The root is less often used but is said to ease a toothache when chewed directly.

Topically, yarrow can be applied to speed up skin healing for dermatitis and lingering skin ailments. The perfect first-aid remedy, the leaves can be applied directly as a poultice to cuts and scrapes, making yarrow the essential herb to forage when out in the wild!

PARTS USED

Flowering tops, leaves, less commonly the root

ENERGETICS

Warming, aromatic, pungent, harmonising, adaptive

ACTIONS

Antihaemorrhagic, anti-inflammatory, antimicrobial, antipyretic, antispasmodic, astringent, bitter tonic, diaphoretic, hemostatic, peripheral vasodilator, styptic, vulnerary

CAUTIONS

Not to be used during lactation; caution with use during pregnancy.

Plants for the People

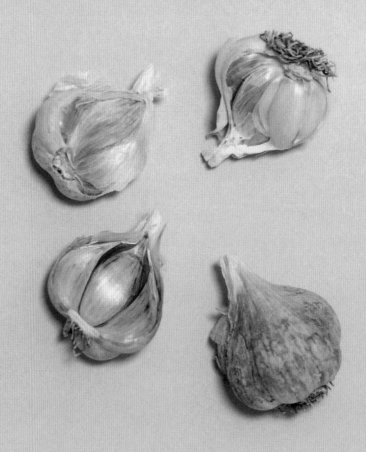

GOLDEN TIP

Avoid odourless capsules –
allow the stinky medicinal
glory of garlic to truly work
its wonders!

ALLIUM SATIVUM
GARLIC

We are all so used to the common name of *Allium sativum*: garlic. But over the ages there have been a bunch of imaginative names for this potent bulb, such as stinking rose, Russian penicillin and poor man's treacle. Garlic is essentially a protector. From historical use by the ancient Greeks to ward off evil spirits to its pop-culture role in guarding against vampires, we have valued this hero bulb for so long that it is hard to trace its origins.

Today, garlic has a prized place in the kitchen and medicine cabinet, and no wonder: not only is it delicious, it is exceptionally mineral and amino-acid dense – basically, really, really good for you! When the clove is crushed, the superpowered constituent alliin transforms into allicin, with hundreds of sulphur-dense compounds, so be sure to always crush your fresh garlic for extra strength.

Garlic is a prime plant medicine for antibiotic-resistant bugs, peptic ulcers (to eradicate *Helicobacter pylori)*, parasitic and bacterial conditions (such as small-intestinal bacterial overgrowth), fungal infections, candida and worms. A supreme immune stimulator, garlic is exceptional at fighting the common cold, hayfever, bronchial congestion, catarrh and influenza, thanks to its mucus-moving, antimicrobial, virus-clearing profile.

With today's epidemic of poor diets and stressed lives, garlic aids the cardiovascular system, reducing and normalising cholesterol levels, decreasing high blood pressure and alleviating atherosclerosis. You can even use garlic cloves or garlic-infused oil topically on angry skin presentations, and fungal and bacterial infections. The aroma may deter your peers, but it will absolutely begin to bust the germs.

Plants for the People

PARTS USED

Bulb, cloves

ENERGETICS

Warming, spicy, yang, drying

ACTIONS

Anthelmintic, antiatherosclerotic, antibacterial, antifungal, antilipidemic, antimicrobial, antioxidant, antiparasitic, antiplatelet, antiprotozoal, antiseptic (gastrointestinal tract), antiviral, carminative, chemoprotective, diuretic, hypocholesterolemic, hypotensive, mucolytic, vasodilator

CAUTIONS

Cease medicinal doses at least 10 days prior to surgery due to blood-thinning properties. Not to be used with anticoagulant prescription medications. Nursing mammas: be mindful that the potency of garlic will flow through your milk to the bambino, potentially contributing to digestive upsets.

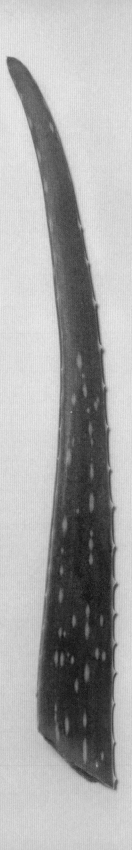

GOLDEN TIP

Aloe vera pulp (made from the
inner gel) added to smoothies
can be lovely and soothing
to the belly, aid gentle toxin
clearance in the liver and boost
the skin to shine.

ALOE BARBADENSIS
ALOE VERA

A tropical succulent beloved for on-the-spot use for all sorts of injuries. Originating in North Africa, this easy-to-cultivate plant has a plethora of medicinal powers. Aloe looks like a spiky, green prehistoric creature, but is way gentler than it may appear. You will spot this low-maintenance plant out and about in many locations. Like all succulents, it can flourish from a simple clipping or root division, and transform into a hearty established plant with time.

Aloe vera is most well known for the mucilaginous inner gel of the leaf. This is commonly applied to the skin to soothe and heal burns, cuts, rashes and abrasions. The gooey gel is at its best fresh – simply slice a leaf open and gently scoop out the jelly from the centre. If you have ever had a scrape and slathered it with the gel of the fresh-cut leaf, you will know the soothing cool and relief it brings. Aloe's wound-healing properties are impressive. It can also be used for reactive skin conditions, such as psoriasis, to ease irritation and inflammation.

Different parts of the aloe plant impact different systems in the body. Taken orally, aloe vera latex (the yellow lining under the plant's skin) has a more marked impact on the digestive system, aiding sluggish elimination, and can be quite purgative due to the anthraquinone action, while the gel is particularly helpful in healing gastric ulcers and stimulating the bowel. It also balances insulin and cholesterol. Wonderful for home beauty recipes, aloe not only hydrates but also stimulates dermal collagen and elastin production for glowy youthfulness.

PARTS USED

Inner gel, latex, whole leaf

ENERGETICS

Bitter, cooling, stimulating, soothing

ACTIONS

Alterative, anthelmintic, anti-inflammatory, antimicrobial (topical), antioxidant (topical), cholagogue, choleretic, collagen synthesiser, immune stimulating (topical), laxative, purgative, stomachic, vulnerary

CAUTIONS

The cautions apply to the use of the inner gel and latex when taken orally – not to topical usage.

Mindful caution during pregnancy and lactation, and for children under the age of twelve. Contraindicated for those with ulcerative colitis and Crohn's disease. Be wise: check interactions with medications. Aloe is best taken orally only for very short periods of time as it can be quite depleting on the systems of the body with extended use.

Plants for the People

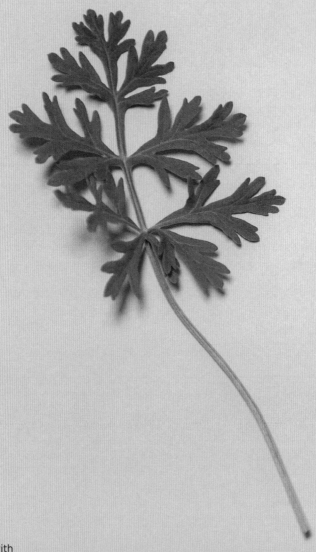

<u>GOLDEN TIP</u>

In combination with other antiparasitics and antimicrobials, such as garlic and thyme, wormwood can drop a loving bomb on a dysbiotic gut, causing the bugs to retreat.

ARTEMISIA ABSINTHIUM
WORMWOOD

A delicate leaf that packs a punch, wormwood is a genuinely ancient plant, popping up in stories from Greek mythology to the Prohibition. Associated with the goddess of wilderness and childbirth, Artemis (also known as Diana), *Artemisia* species have historically been associated with birthing in many facets. Wormwood holds a potent constituent, thujone, within its silverish leaves. Thujone is responsible for the plant's hallucinatory action in absinthe, the notorious bitter liqueur that was popular during the 19th century, before being banned for almost a hundred years. Please be assured it takes mammoth amounts of wormwood (which would be hazardous to ingest) to get close to the side effects of this historical concoction.

Today, we value wormwood for the digestive system particularly, specifically to clear parasitic and worm-fuelled intestinal overgrowths – think pinworm or roundworm. It stimulates digestion, addressing low stomach acid, nausea, bloating and colic. There is a uterine-stimulating element, which ties into the historical use for labouring women. It is absolutely to be avoided during pregnancy due to this mechanism! Wormwood is also a potent easer of fevers, colds and flus. It is likely the most bitter herb out there, perhaps a little challenging on the palate, but if this can be overcome, it is a valuable stimulator of digestion, improving appetite when taken before a meal. Bottoms up!

PARTS USED

Flowers, leaves

ENERGETICS

Cooling, bitter, awakening, stimulating, defender

ACTIONS

Anthelmintic, antibacterial, antifungal, anti-inflammatory, antimalarial, antiparasitic, antiseptic (gastrointestinal tract), aromatic, bitter tonic, choleretic, emmenagogue, expectorant, febrifuge, neuroprotective, stomachic

CAUTIONS

Avoid prolonged use: aim to limit use to short periods of time – 3 weeks maximum. Avoid during pregnancy and breastfeeding, and with ulcerations of the gastrointestinal tract.

Plants for the People

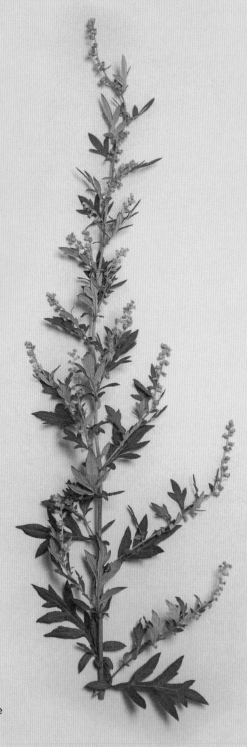

GOLDEN TIP

When making mugwort tea, be sure to brew with a lid on to trap the beneficial volatile oils. Follow a shorter brew time as this is one strong aromatic plant! Complement with sweeter herbs to round out the underlying bitterness mugwort may bring to the tastebuds.

ARTEMISIA VULGARIS
MUGWORT

Mugwort is a wise wild weed used traditionally by Native Americans as a spiritual and medicinal ally. Leaves were rubbed over the body to repel spirits, or worn as a necklace to promote pleasant dreams. Native American women called upon magical mugwort's emmenagogue powers to bring forth a delayed menstrual cycle. This traditional knowledge has set a precedent for mugwort's mystical and practical applications.

Today we look to mugwort to regulate a stagnated, heavy or delayed menstrual cycle, to bring warmth to the womb. There is also an incredible mechanism within the medicine of mugwort that amplifies prophetic dream realms. Pop a small handful of dried mugwort or fresh leaf in a little muslin bag, keep it close by your pillow and see how your dream states shift!

There is a calming air to mugwort, providing support for anxiety, insomnia and depression, and settling reactive bellies, while the aromatic bitter attributes of the plant gently stimulate the liver and digestion. Much like its relative wormwood, mugwort also expels intestinal infestations (think worms and parasites).

Mugwort continues to play an important part in ceremony in many traditions, aiding shamanic journeys and being burnt for protection, clearing and blessings.

PARTS USED

Leaves, flowers, rarely the root

ENERGETICS

Warming, bitter, acrid

ACTIONS

Anthelmintic, antiseptic, antispasmodic, bitter tonic, choleretic, emmenagogue, oneirogen, orexigenic, stomachic, uterine tonic

CAUTIONS

Avoid during pregnancy and lactation.

Plants for the People

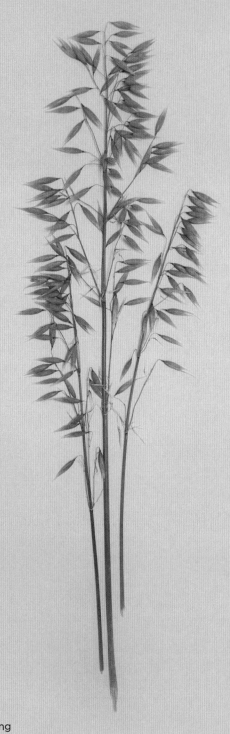

GOLDEN TIP

A bowl of whole oat porridge
is food as medicine at its
best, promoting bowel flow
with fibre-dense goodness,
balancing blood sugar levels,
aiding heart health and lowering
cholesterol with beta-glucans.

AVENA SATIVA
OATS

Whole oats are synonymous with a wholesome breakfast – and rightly so, as they hold a treasure chest of cosiness and nourishment within their little husks. In the herbal realms, this ancient grain contains a whole lot of mighty medicine. It is such a versatile plant: the young milky green tops are commonly used, as are the dried stems we refer to as oat straw. Oat straw and milky oats vary slightly in their profiles, but I will address the wonderful *Avena sativa* more generally here. This nutrient-dense powerhouse is particularly rich in silica, iron, manganese, B vitamins and zinc, so the way we have traditionally used oats – cooking and eating them to warm and fill a hungry belly – makes complete sense.

The medicine of oats ties into the satiety they bring: a steaming bowl of porridge will stoke the fire within, much as oats do for the nervous system. They stabilise and replenish a deeper hunger, filling a depleted, distracted, exhausted, nervous person with warmth and restoration. The spirit of oats is captured perfectly by the term 'trophorestorative', which is what we herbalists call a herb that is suitable for longer-term use to rebuild and restore the energy of a particular system. *Avena sativa* is a trophorestorative for the nervous system, and a true tonic for the frayed, depressed, anxious, insomnia stricken, stressed, overstretched and traumatised, repairing burnt-out adrenal energy. Oats are incredible for those convalescing or combating recurring outbreaks of herpes virus strains, such as cold sores and shingles. Adding whole oats to a warm bath (in a stocking or muslin bag) creates a soothing milky pool in which to immerse dry, itchy, irritated skin – a great calming remedy for eczema.

Oats offer us strength when we are journeying through challenging territories.

PARTS USED

Seeds, tops, leaves, stems

ENERGETICS

Sweet, nutritive, warming, neutral, soothing

ACTIONS

Alterative, antidepressant, antihypertensive, anti-inflammatory, antilipidemic, antipruritic, emollient, hypoglycaemic, nervine tonic, sedative, thymoleptic, tonic, trophorestorative, vulnerary

CAUTIONS

Caution with use in coeliac disease and if you are exceptionally sensitive to gluten.

Plants for the People

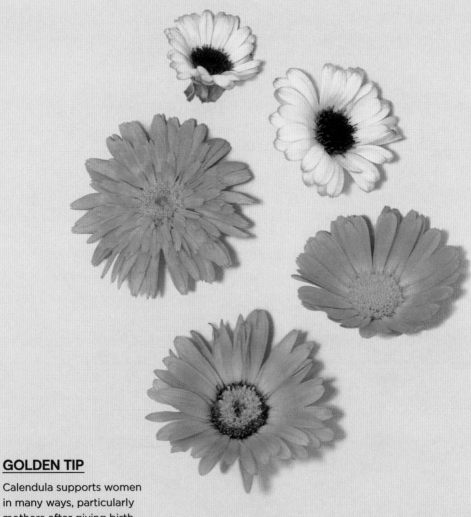

GOLDEN TIP

Calendula supports women
in many ways, particularly
mothers after giving birth.
A sitz bath (essentially a
giant tea bath) can be made
with the dried flower heads.
Mamma can immerse her
pelvis in the warm infused
water to heal, soothe and
restore tissues.

CALENDULA OFFICINALIS
CALENDULA

A hardy, classic European plant, calendula is a beacon of herbal sunshine that on many levels embodies the energy of sunrays. It is astrologically connected to the forces of the sun and appears like a luminous sea of yellow and orange beams when in bloom. This plant medicine is an amateur gardener's delight: no fuss and low maintenance, responding to harvest of the flower heads by growing more with abundance.

Cheerful calendula alleviates melancholy and stagnation, making it a wonderful ally for those feeling low and in need of a lift. Kin to the lymphatic system, calendula is an impeccable remedy for any lymphatic congestion, such as swollen glands, acne and cysts. It has a warming effect internally, aiding clearance within the lymphatic, hepatic and gastrointestinal organ systems to shift underlying stasis. Calendula supports detoxification and releases an overburdened liver. Digestively, it is wonderful for irritable bowel syndrome, food allergies and intolerances, leaky gut syndrome and inflammatory bowel disease. There is also a hormone-balancing element to calendula, specific to normalising irregular menstrual cycles and calming painful menstruation.

Beyond these plentiful indications, calendula really shines with topical use, the golden flowers encouraging tissue and cellular regeneration. Use on burns, cuts, ulcers, acne, eczema, dermatitis, bites, varicose veins, nappy rash, haemorrhoids, bruises and skin infections. Be it in a balm, oil, mouthwash or infusion, this plant medicine is one to keep handy.

Many consider calendula to have a cooling energy, but overall it radiates a deep, sincere warmth, permeating our systems with a flush of gentle heat. Calendula is an awakener, reminding us to shake off unnecessary burdens and feel the warmth of the sun on our cheeks.

Plants for the People

PARTS USED

Whole flower heads

ENERGETICS

Warming, drying, clearing, freeing, brightening

ACTIONS

Alterative, antifungal, anti-inflammatory, antimicrobial, antiviral, astringent, cholagogue, choleretic, emmenagogue, lymphatic, styptic, vulnerary

CAUTIONS

Avoid use during pregnancy and lactation and if allergic or sensitive to the Asteraceae (daisy) family.

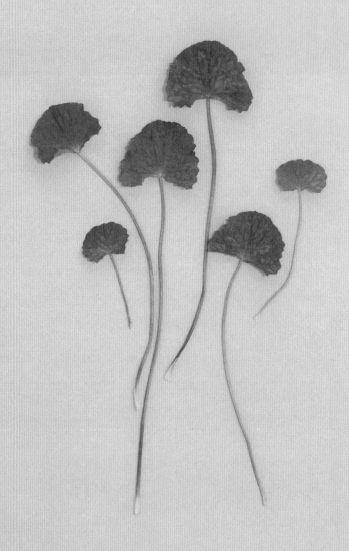

GOLDEN TIP

A fresh poultice of the gotu kola
leaf applied straight to the skin is
the perfect way to cool a burn.

WILD WEED

CENTELLA ASIATICA
GOTU KOLA

Gotu kola is an edible pantropical plant with a penchant for wound healing. Growing prolifically in Australia, Asia, Africa and the Americas, this lawn-loving weed favours damp, humid environments. In Ayurvedic medicine, gotu kola is valued as a prime elixir for restoring vitality and supercharging cognition. Cherished by yogis over the ages, it is revered as a gateway plant for developing the crown chakra and deepening meditation.

Overall, gotu kola is a supreme adaptogenic tonic with the ability to combat a depleted, frenetic state, calm the nervous system and quieten a busy mind. It is the perfect plant medicine to replenish the tank, adapt the stress response and increase endurance and energy. When taken orally, gotu kola supports venous sufficiency and flow, aiding varicose veins, restless legs and arthritis.

A strengthening quality resounds in all applications of this powerful herbal ally, due to its ability to stimulate collagen synthesis. It is even indicated to strengthen and promote hair, nail and skin growth. Topically, it is a superstar wound healer used to prevent scar tissue formation after surgery, speed up healing in wounds, ulcerations, burns, psoriasis and varicose veins, and much more.

Gotu kola gives us a clue to another application in its appearance, resembling a brain: there are two distinct sides to the leaf, representing the left and right hemispheres. It offers up soft yin energy to balance our busy brains and enhance longevity, and sharpens memory with its antioxidant-rich regenerative powers.

PARTS USED

Leaves, less often roots

ENERGETICS

Bitter, cooling, sweet, reparative

ACTIONS

Adaptogenic, alterative, antifibrotic, anti-inflammatory, antioxidant, connective-tissue regenerator, immunomodulator, nervine, neuroregenerative, neuroprotective, vulnerary

CAUTIONS

Caution with use during pregnancy. Avoid if allergic to the Apiaceae (carrot) family.

Plants for the People

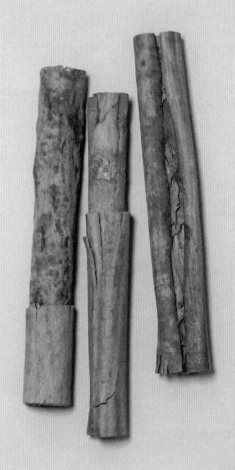

GOLDEN TIP

Cinnamon is a great way to
sweeten porridge, smoothies
and tonics without adding
an extra sugary element. Try
pairing it with vanilla powder –
this combo sweetens, warms,
lifts and lightens.

CINNAMOMUM CASSIA, CINNAMOMUM VERUM
CINNAMON

The essence of warmth is wrapped within the rolled bark of cinnamon. This is the plant for restoring the fire within, replenishing vitality and stimulating energy flow throughout the body. A classic traditional Chinese medicine, cinnamon is a true plant of the East, one of the first to be traded via the spice routes from Sri Lanka to the Middle East.

Think of cinnamon as an overall tonic for the body: it has a systemic impact, flushing our beings with sweetness. It gives us that little nudge to spark the light if it has been too dim lately.

Physically, cinnamon has a range of applications. The bark balances blood sugar levels, warms blood flow to the uterus, alleviates the common cold, relieves digestive spasms, eases loose stools, reduces a gassy belly, calms nausea and stimulates the appetite. This is a stand-out herbal medicine to apply frequently for diabetes, insulin resistance and syndrome X, and a wise, accessible spice to weave into your daily rhythms.

PARTS USED

Inner bark, stems

ENERGETICS

Warming, sweet, hot, spicy, rejuvenating

ACTIONS

Antidiabetic, antidiarrhoeal, antifungal, antimicrobial, antiseptic, antispasmodic, antiviral, astringent, carminative, circulatory stimulant, digestive, hypocholesterolemic, hypoglycaemic, mucolytic

CAUTIONS

Avoid use during pregnancy, or with stomach or duodenal ulcerations.

Plants for the People

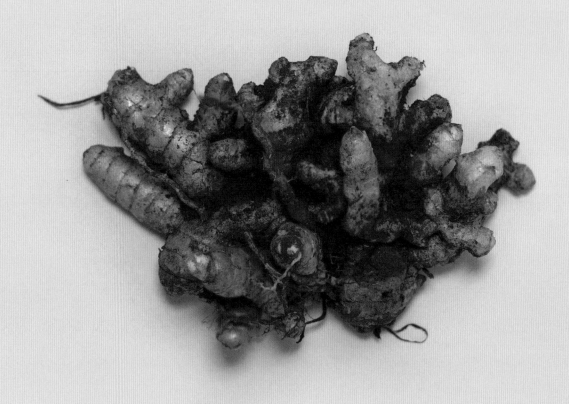

GOLDEN TIP

Curcumin is the star
compound in the plant; to
enhance bioavailability and
absorbability, pair with black
pepper (rich in piperine) and
a beneficial fat, such as ghee.

CURCUMA LONGA
TURMERIC

The benefits of this golden-yellow rhizome have long been hailed in the East; in more recent times, love for turmeric has ignited in the West too. Preferring to grow in balmy climates, turmeric is a finger-like rhizomatous bulb, sprouting beautiful tropical blooms atop lush, green leaves. Closely related to ginger, it belongs to the same family, the Zingiberaceae clan. The gowns of Buddhist monks are often dyed naturally with the bold, beautiful tones of turmeric, dubbed 'Indian saffron'.

We commonly value turmeric as a culinary spice that brings pungency and warmth. However, this is one remarkable medicinal plant, a full-force antioxidant and potent anti-inflammatory. Turmeric is prescribed for its restorative, enhancing actions on the hepatobiliary system, repairing damage, decongesting, and boosting poor function, to shift a sluggish gall bladder and stimulate valuable detoxification phases of the liver. A support for the digestive system, it is wonderful for bellyaches of all sorts, low appetite, nausea, vomiting and overall to aid an under-functioning gut. Indicated to reduce chronic inflammation in many forms, turmeric is known to assist in a lengthy list of conditions: cancers, degenerative neurological diseases such as Alzheimer's, cardiovascular conditions, elevated cholesterol and atherosclerosis, osteoarthritis, rheumatoid arthritis, diabetes, allergies and sensitivities, asthma, inflammatory bowel disease, gastric ulcerations, irritable bowel syndrome, chronic skin conditions, menstrual irregularities, yeast overgrowths...the list goes on and on!

PARTS USED

Rhizome

ENERGETICS

Warming, pungent, drying, spicy

ACTIONS

Alterative, anticancer, anticoagulant, anti-inflammatory, antioxidant, antiplatelet, antiseptic, astringent, cardioprotective, cholerectic, cholagogue, emmenagogue, hepatoprotective, immune enhancing

CAUTIONS

Avoid with bile duct obstruction and with gallstones. Caution with use during pregnancy and lactation. Caution in concomitant use with anticoagulant pharmaceuticals.

Classically, turmeric is thought to have an anti-fertility action, so if you are looking to conceive, shelve this healer for the time being.

Plants for the People

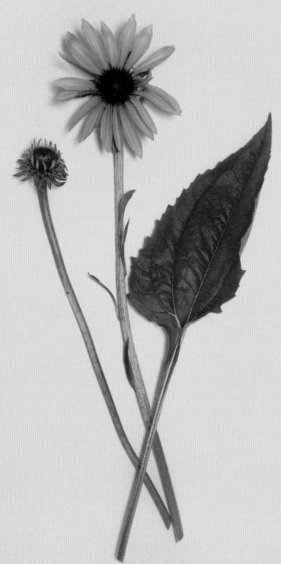

GOLDEN TIP

Echinacea is a sialagogue,
meaning it stimulates your
salivary glands. To test its
potency, taste a little; if your
mouth begins to water and
tingle, you are working with
a good-quality echinacea!

ECHINACEA SPP.
ECHINACEA

There are many species of this beloved native North American plant, the beautiful purple coneflower. The three most commonly cultivated varieties nowadays are *Echinacea angustifolia*, *Echinacea pallida* and *Echinacea purpurea*. Each has unique qualities, but overall, echinacea species are superb immune-enhancing allies that act with might on the lymphatic system.

Traditionally, echinacea played a large part in the Native American apothecary – so much so that it was said to be used for more ailments than any other plant. The ripples of knowledge found their way into the hands of eclectic medicine practitioners – a group of late 19th-century doctors who employed botanical remedies. From here, echinacea wove its way to the forefront of herbal medicine.

The list of uses is lengthy – are you ready? With an affection for the immune system, echinacea is commonly prescribed for viral, bacterial and parasitic infections. It is a powerful remedy for conditions of the upper and lower respiratory systems, combating colds, flus, fevers, pneumonia, conjunctivitis, ear infections, sinusitis, tonsillitis, coughs and bronchitis. With its lymphatic powers, it is a wonderful aid for swollen lymph glands and improves skin conditions such as dermatitis, psoriasis, shingles, herpes, acne and ulcerations. It is often utilised as an adjunct therapy in cancer treatment alongside chemotherapy and radiotherapy. Echinacea also has an affinity for the gastrointestinal system and is indicated in digestive infections, candida, peptic ulcerations and hepatitis. It is a major herbal star for kidney and urinary tract infections. Think of echinacea if you are experiencing chronic fatigue syndrome, fibromyalgia or any chronic post-viral symptoms. Topically, it is also an excellent wound healer.

The energy of echinacea is like a trusted friend showing up with a pot of soup when you are under the weather, to lift your spirits and get you on the road to recovery. What can't this plant do?

PARTS USED

Roots predominantly, also seeds, flowers, leaves

ENERGETICS

Cooling, sweet, drying, warming, stimulating

ACTIONS

Alterative, antibacterial, antifungal, anti-inflammatory, antimicrobial, antiseptic, antiviral, depurative, diaphoretic, immune enhancing, immunomodulator, lymphatic, sialagogue, vasodilator, vulnerary

CAUTIONS

Asthmatics and those with autoimmune conditions should exercise caution. Also, for anyone who has allergies to the Asteraceae (daisy) family, avoid!

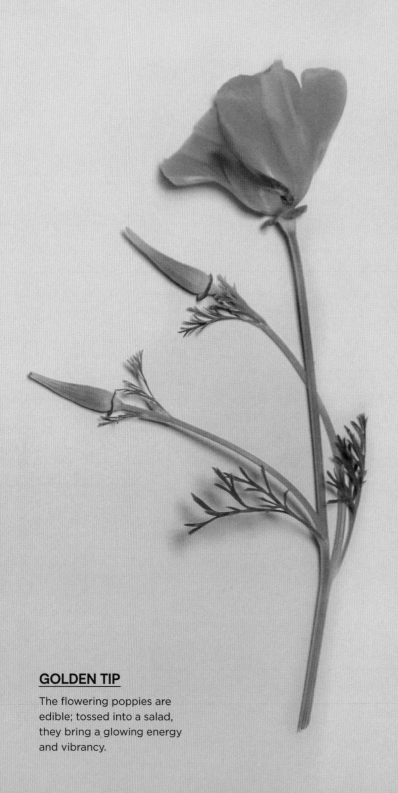

GOLDEN TIP

The flowering poppies are
edible; tossed into a salad,
they bring a glowing energy
and vibrancy.

ESCHSCHOLZIA CALIFORNICA
CALIFORNIAN POPPY

Californian poppy is a wildflower native to North America. When the stars align, a breathtaking spring super-bloom blankets the rugged coastline of California, covering hills and terrain in a sea of orange. Spanish settlers sailing into the headlands called California the 'land of fire' due to the poppies lighting up the landscape. Although this cheery poppy is not the most common outside of America, it is incredibly garden friendly and easy to grow in varied conditions.

Californian poppy has long been an important herbal medicine in Native American traditions, used to alleviate toothaches and physical pains, and not much has changed in the way we work with this plant medicine. It is an outstanding reliever of all types of nerve-related pains, such as neuralgia, shingles, toothaches, headaches, menstrual cramps and sciatica.

Californian poppy has a marked sedative action, providing aid for insomnia, anxiety, panic attacks, emotional stress and sensitive, hyperactive nervous systems. Like the opium poppy, there are alkaloids present in the plant – minus the opiates – so it's much gentler, safer and non-addictive. You can expect a feeling of tranquillity, like listening to a soft lullaby, when connecting to the medicine of this plant.

PARTS USED

Flowers, leaves, seeds, roots

ENERGETICS

Cooling, bitter, relaxing

ACTIONS

Analgesic, anodyne, antispasmodic, anxiolytic, hypnotic, nervine, sedative

CAUTIONS

Avoid combining with any pain-relieving or sedative pharmaceuticals. Avoid during breastfeeding and pregnancy, and use with caution for pain in children.

Plants for the People

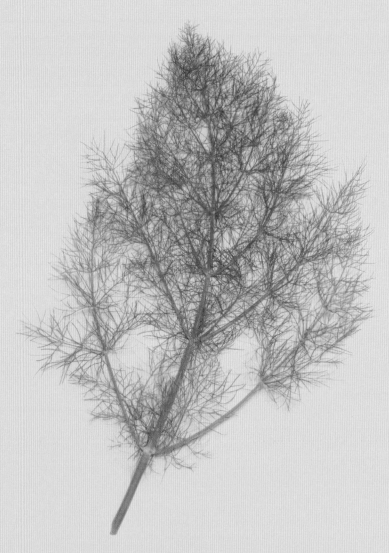

GOLDEN TIP

Fennel seeds in combination
with raw honey make a
delicious infused syrup
that is particularly helpful
for persistent coughs and
respiratory congestion.

WILD WEED

FOENICULUM VULGARE
FENNEL

Hailing from the Mediterranean, fennel is now naturalised and cultivated worldwide. In Australia and North America, you will find these wild weeds lining roadsides, graceful and tall, their seed heads blooming in a yellow flurry of colour. Fennel is an age-old remedy, used medicinally in the Middle Ages and as far back as the ancient Greeks and Romans, who believed it bestowed courage, longevity and strength.

Fennel has an aromatic quality with a warm aniseed flavour. The small seeds are often chewed directly to soothe a reactive belly and freshen the breath. Fennel is akin to the digestive system, easing all sorts of uncomfortable symptoms such as bloating, nausea, gas, indigestion and intestinal spasms, and a true friend to those who experience irritable bowel syndrome symptoms. The seed is often used for bronchial afflictions, asthma, coughs and catarrh, and an eyewash can be made to combat conjunctivitis. There is a hormone-balancing power to fennel, alleviating amenorrhoea and dysmenorrhoea, while having a slight oestrogenic effect – hence why large amounts are cautioned against during pregnancy. However, fennel is a true companion for new mammas, easing infantile intestinal colic and encouraging a mother's milk supply with its supportive galactagogue action.

For such a common wild weed, there is really nothing common about it!

PARTS USED

Fruits, seeds

ENERGETICS

Warming, spicy, drying, sweet

ACTIONS

Anti-inflammatory, antimicrobial, antispasmodic, aromatic, carminative, expectorant, galactagogue, oestrogen modulator, orexigenic, stimulant

CAUTIONS

During pregnancy, be sure to avoid large amounts.

Plants for the People

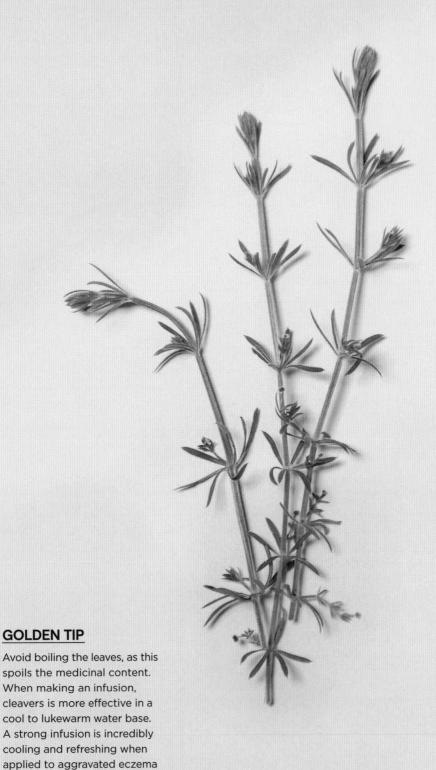

GOLDEN TIP

Avoid boiling the leaves, as this spoils the medicinal content. When making an infusion, cleavers is more effective in a cool to lukewarm water base. A strong infusion is incredibly cooling and refreshing when applied to aggravated eczema or overheated, sunburnt skin.

GALIUM APARINE
CLEAVERS

With distinctive fine hairs along the stems, cleavers manages to cling to all it touches, living up to its nickname 'stickyweed'. This is actually how the wild weed manages to spread itself so prolifically, catching a ride in the wind and on animals, people and fellow plants, embodying the energy of adaptation and survival. It blooms in spring, much like we do, awakening from winter's slumber, and is valued for its blood-cleansing and diuretic effect, purifying and ushering out the stagnancy within our systems – just what is needed after the inward energy of winter months.

An impressive lymphatic tonifier with the ability to speak directly to glandular congestion, cleavers is a prime remedy for shifting swollen glands and nodes. As with any plant akin to the lymphatic system, there is a strong indication for use in all forms of chronic skin disorders, making cleavers a wonderful ally to improve acne, eczema, psoriasis, rosacea and urticaria. As a fresh poultice, it brings cooling relief for growths, cysts, acne, boils, abscesses, sunburn, wounds and blisters, counteracting red, reactive, sore, stuck, slow-healing states. The bladder and kidneys respond with positivity to this wild weed, which soothes and alleviates fluid retention while restoring the flow within the organ systems.

Cleavers brings spring cleansing and cooling to our bodies in a way that is gentle and sustainable for longer-term use, offering a more sustained energy for the people. You will most likely find this plant growing nearby and abundantly, as it has made itself a home worldwide. Connect with cleavers' medicine in early spring just as it awakens and the flowers begin to blossom.

Plants for the People

PARTS USED

Leaves, flowers, stems, full aerial parts

CAUTIONS

None known.

ENERGETICS

Fresh, cooling, drying, rejuvenating

ACTIONS

Alterative, anti-inflammatory, antispasmodic, astringent, depurative, diuretic, lymphatic

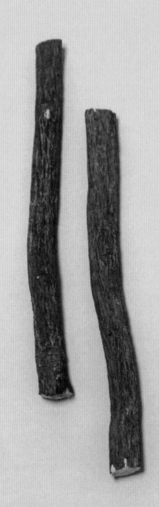

GOLDEN TIP

Licorice will sweeten even
the most heinous-tasting
herbal formulas – a trick we
herbalists employ on the daily!

GLYCYRRHIZA GLABRA
LICORICE

Licorice is curiously complex and marvellously medicinal. In my opinion it is one of the most relevant plant medicines for the modern day. Our emotions and environments play a huge role in our physical health; particularly impacted are our hypersensitive endocrine systems, responsible for our hormonal harmony. We live in a mighty yang world, full of doing and the glorification of busyness. Women especially deeply feel this, and our hormones reflect it all. Burnout, exhaustion, hypothalamic-pituitary-adrenal (HPA) axis disorders, adrenal fatigue, adrenal depletion, chronic fatigue syndrome and fibromyalgia are a confronting reality for many, alongside hormonal imbalances such as premenstrual tension, irregular menstrual cycles, polycystic ovarian syndrome (PCOS), endometriosis, androgen excess and infertility. Licorice is a light for adrenally depleted folk, a sweet adaptogenic elixir of restoration. It recalibrates the adrenal glands, reduces the symptoms of androgen dominance so prevalent in PCOS presentations, and addresses imbalanced blood sugar levels, which is key for happy hormones.

Demulcent in nature, licorice soothes, coats and protects the respiratory and gastrointestinal systems, relieving colds, asthma, bronchial congestion and coughs, while exerting immune-modulating, antiviral and antibacterial powers. An anti-inflammatory force for the mucous membranes of the gut, licorice assists in gastritis, peptic and duodenal ulcerations, reflux, constipation and irritable bowel syndrome, while supporting the healthy function of the liver, kidneys and bladder. Generally indicated for inflammatory skin conditions when applied topically, this sweet root delivers a moistening action, alleviating dry, irritated states.

In truth, the list of its medicinal wisdoms could go on and on. Licorice embodies regeneration – consider this herbal superstar to build up your vitality, strength and energy stores if they are feeling a little (or a lot) lacklustre.

PARTS USED

Roots

ENERGETICS

Warming, pungent, sweet, nutritious

ACTIONS

Adaptogenic, adrenal modulator, anti-inflammatory, antiseptic (urinary system), antispasmodic (uterus), antitussive, antiulcerogenic (gastrointestinal tract), antiviral (topical), aperient, demulcent, expectorant, hypoglycaemic, mucoprotective, oestrogenic

CAUTIONS

Avoid during pregnancy and lactation. Steer clear if fluid retention, hypertension, heart disease, low potassium states, liver conditions or kidney disorders are present. Elderly people with pre-existing conditions of the kidneys, heart or liver, and men with low testosterone levels, should use with caution.

Plants for the People

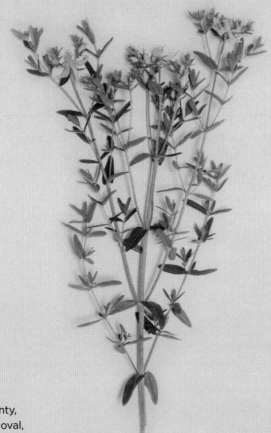

GOLDEN TIP

To identify with certainty,
hold one of the small, oval,
veined leaves up to the light;
you should see pinprick-
like perforations (hence the
species name, *perforatum*).
Another easy approach is to
pick the brilliant yellow flower
or bud and squeeze between
your fingers – a red stain
should be excreted; this is the
colour of one of the active
constituents, hypericin.

WILD WEED

HYPERICUM PERFORATUM
ST JOHN'S WORT

Gloriously cheerful St John's wort is native to Europe, Asia and North Africa and has naturalised in North America and Australia. It grows abundantly in the wild and is mostly found in drought-tolerant pastures, farmland, trails and gravelly, rich soils. With its five-petalled, bright-yellow flowers popping in early to full summer, it is hard to miss!

This striking herbaceous perennial has been utilised as a healing plant from the time of the ancient Greeks through to the Middle Ages, and in Native American traditional medicine. The common name is derived from the date of flowering and harvesting in the northern hemisphere, around 24 June, St John's Day. Historically, St John's wort was thought of as a mystical plant, imbibed to protect against the dark forces and to promote good fortune. It was used for wound healing, soothing bites, nervous tension, depression, ulcerations and to ease a myriad of physical pains.

Brilliantly, our modern use of St John's wort mirrors the historical applications; nowadays it is ubiquitous as an emotional health support. Heavily researched for its impact on depression and anxiety, this plant shines as a remedy for burnout, exhaustion and fatigue. With a true affinity for the nervous system, St John's wort eases neuropathic pain and has a marked effect on herpes viruses, such as cold sores and shingles.

PARTS USED

Flowers, leaves, stems – the upper aerial parts

ENERGETICS

Sunny, supportive, uplifting, stabilising, pungent

ACTIONS

Anodyne, antidepressant, anti-inflammatory, antiseptic (topically), antiviral, anxiolytic, astringent, cholagogue, digestive, hepatoprotective, nervine, relaxant, trophorestorative, vulnerary

CAUTIONS

Not to be used during pregnancy or lactation. Avoid excessive sunlight while using St John's wort due to its ability to cause photosensitivity. St John's wort is contraindicated with multiple pharmaceutical medications, including the oral contraceptive pill and many antidepressants, such as SSRIs – please do your research!

Plants for the People

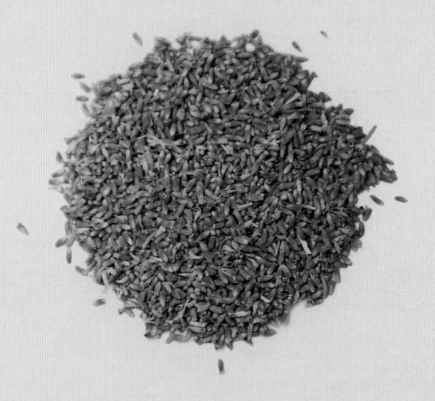

<u>GOLDEN TIP</u>

Lavender pairs synergistically
with chamomile; taken as a
loose-leaf tea or combined in a
herbal bath, these floral healers
bring a soothing serenity.

LAVANDULA ANGUSTIFOLIA
LAVENDER

Indigenous to the Mediterranean, lavender provides cooling relief, melting away tension. The name itself brings a sensory reaction if one is familiar with the scent. Lavender evokes sweet dreams and eases a frayed nervous system. A noble anxiolytic, it sedates an edgy mind and body, making it the perfect plant medicine to ease stress, nervousness, insomnia, anxiety and headaches. There is an uplifting spirit permeating the lilac-coloured buds, which offer a helping hand for mild depression and are particularly in tune with women and menopausal folk. Lavender soothes the belly, relieving digestive cramping and spasms. The oil is renowned for its heavenly fragrance and relaxing properties, and is therapeutically equipped with a bounty of topical applications, from sunburn relief to insect bite treatment.

   Lavender has a strong relationship to ritual and has been called upon over the ages for love, peace and protection. There is a gentleness in lavender that aligns with the energy of little ones, allowing newborns, infants and children to respond well to the aroma. Lavender offers us all the opportunity to lean in to its sweet floral bouquet.

PARTS USED

Flowers

ENERGETICS

Cooling, relaxing, drying, uplifting

ACTIONS

Analgesic (mild), anticonvulsant, antidepressant, antimicrobial, antioxidant, antispasmodic (muscles), anxiolytic, carminative, sedative, stomachic

CAUTIONS

Caution with concomitant use with pharmaceutical antidepressants. Best avoided during pregnancy.

Plants for the People

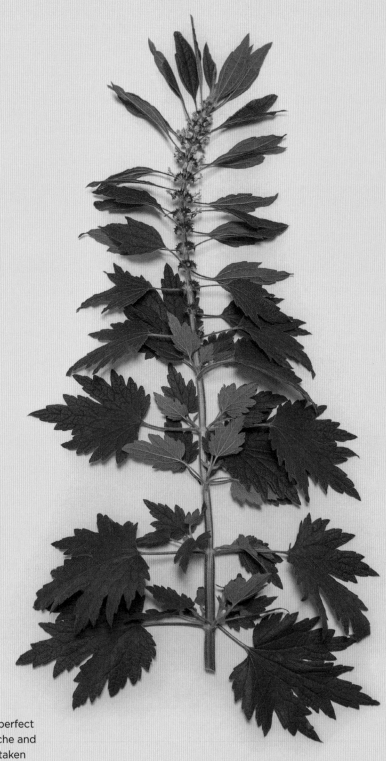

GOLDEN TIP

Motherwort is the perfect
remedy for heartache and
heartbreak – even taken
as a flower essence it is
supportive and reparative.

LEONURUS CARDIACA
MOTHERWORT

With some of the best known common names around, motherwort (aka the lion-hearted, lion's tale, lion's ear, heartwort, throw-wort) is a plant with a firm place in herbal healing over the ages. Indigenous to Europe and Asia, and naturalised in North America, this is a wild weed in the eyes of many. Like any relative of the sprawling mints, growth can be prolific and a little unkempt.

Motherwort expresses a matriarchal energy of care and comfort, a safe harbour in which to take shelter. It is the perfect plant remedy to ease anxiety, emotional burnout, melancholy and depression, with an invocation of peace woven within the field of its medicine. Not only does it lift the heart and drive away the blues, motherwort also has an affinity for some cardiovascular symptoms, such as irregular heartbeats, palpitations and nervous tachycardia (speedy heartbeat). This makes motherwort an incredible ally to regulate hyperthyroidism, where heart palpitations aplenty often occur. For ovarian pain or a missing, stagnant or overzealous menstrual cycle, motherwort is indicated to encourage regulation and hormonal support. It is a key herb for use in menopause, addressing not only physical manifestations but also the emotional landscape as a woman transitions from mother to crone.

Think of motherwort as a much-needed warm, settling embrace to combat excess energy of the heart and mind, full of earthy nourishment and serene forces.

PARTS USED

Leaves, flowers

ENERGETICS

Maternal, drying, cooling, relaxing

ACTIONS

Analgesic (mild), antiarrhythmic, antidepressant, antispasmodic (uterus), antithyroid, astringent, cardiotonic, emmenagogue, hypotensive, nervine, sedative, spasmolytic, uterine stimulant, uterine tonic

CAUTIONS

Avoid use during pregnancy, due to the uterine-stimulating properties. Contraindicated in those with hypothyroid symptoms or pathology. Caution with regular use in endometriosis and where uterine fibroids are present.

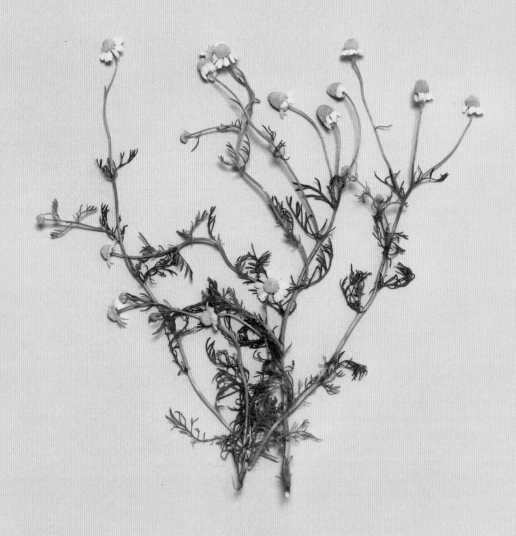

GOLDEN TIP

The perfect cup of tea post
dinner, chamomile aids
digestion while soothing the
nerves to unwind for a night of
sound sleep. It is said to induce
nothing but sweet dreams!

MATRICARIA CHAMOMILLA
CHAMOMILE (GERMAN)

One of the softest energies of the plant medicine kingdom, chamomile has a sweet, easy nature. It has long been held in sacred regard – so much so that some cultures bow to the plant when passing by. It is easy to understand: there is something a little mystical in the perfection of chamomile, from the delicate white-petalled, yellow-centred flowers to its intoxicating sweet-smelling foliage. Chamomile is a deep exhale for the nervous system, specifically for restlessness, irritability and sensitivity.

Therapeutically, chamomile's yin-like energy is particularly suited to women and children, and the inner child within us all. It is a very safe and easy-to-use plant; simply drinking it as a tea can bring much-needed serenity. Wonderful for teething infants, it is a top choice among many herbalists for alleviating the challenges associated with cutting teeth. Chamomile calms digestive concerns such as indigestion, bloating, gastritis, diarrhoea and motion sickness by easing intestinal spasms, healing gastric ulcerations and soothing an anxious belly.

Topically, chamomile has a wound-healing effect; a simple infusion can be applied to dermatitis, ulcerations and wounds. Our immune systems also respond beautifully to chamomile, which provides relief for asthma, colds, fevers, influenza and seasonal allergies.

Truly this plant is a heal-all, with so many indications that the list could go on and on. Primarily, however, think of this petite daisy-like flower for anxiety, insomnia and weary nervous systems that are in dire need of a break.

PARTS USED

Flowers

ENERGETICS

Sweet, bitter, harmonising

ACTIONS

Analgesic, antiallergic, anticatarrhal, anti-inflammatory, antimicrobial, antiseptic, antispasmodic, antiulcerogenic (gastrointestinal tract), carminative, cholagogue, diaphoretic, digestive, emmenagogue, nervine, sedative (mild), vulnerary

CAUTIONS

Avoid in known allergy to Asteraceae (daisy) family.

Plants for the People

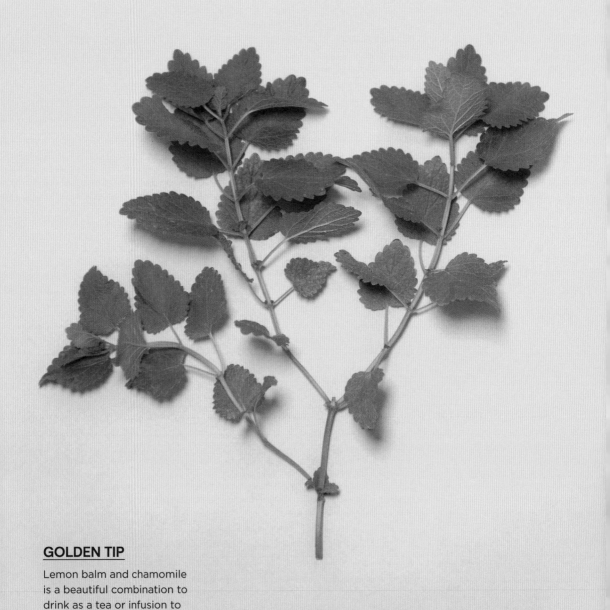

GOLDEN TIP

Lemon balm and chamomile
is a beautiful combination to
drink as a tea or infusion to
soothe the nerves and calm
the belly.

MELISSA OFFICINALIS
LEMON BALM

Lemon balm is a member of the mint family, which is a direct clue to how it grows – with great ease! Historically, this classic European and Mediterranean herb was used by kings and queens and affectionately dubbed the 'herbal cure-all'. Ancient Greeks and Romans noted its medicinal applications, and an Arabic proverb is said to have stated: 'Balm makes the heart merry and joyful.'

The ancient ones understood the beautiful lemon balm; it truly embodies the calming, uplifting forces plants can offer us all. There is a sweetness, an inherent femininity to this plant. Lemon balm has a fortifying energy, promoting relaxation and soothing the unsettled. This applies to upset bellies, overactive thyroids, viral expressions, colds, fevers, anxiety, insomnia, headaches, depression, hypertension and neuralgia.

Lemon balm is a key herb for irritable bowel syndrome. The symptoms of this condition (bloating, gas, changeable stools) often stem from a stress-induced response, the classic presentation of a nervous gut – and lemon balm is wonderful for all stress-related symptoms. It turns down the intensity with ease and grace. Applied topically, it has a strong antiviral action, wonderful for cold sores and relevant all round for herpes viruses. Lemon balm is a gentle, effective herb to use for little ones experiencing colic and digestive upsets. Unlike many other herbal remedies, lemon balm has a really pleasant taste and is just perfect picked from the garden for a medicinal brew.

PARTS USED

Leaves

ENERGETICS

Calming, pungent, cooling

ACTIONS

Antimicrobial, antioxidant, antipyretic, antispasmodic (muscles), antiviral, carminative, diaphoretic, emmenagogue, nervine, sedative, stomachic, TSH antagonist

CAUTIONS

Lemon balm is generally an exceptionally safe plant, but please practise caution during pregnancy and with hypothyroidism.

Plants for the People

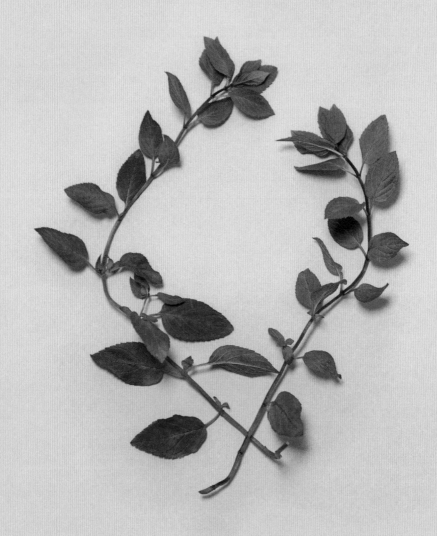

GOLDEN TIP

In combination with
chamomile buds, peppermint
makes the perfect tea for a
child's upset belly.

MENTHA X PIPERITA
PEPPERMINT

Peppermint is said to be a hybrid, born from the evolution of water mint and spearmint – a plant medicine holding the wisdom of the mints within. It has a lengthy history of medicinal use dating back to the ancient Egyptians, although it rose to fame over the past few centuries as an exceptional stomach soother.

Peppermint speaks to the digestive system with a calming tone. This plant medicine reduces tumultuous gas in the belly, making it the most fitting remedy for colic, flatulence and irritable bowel syndrome symptoms. It has a direct antispasmodic effect on the smooth muscle tissue of the gastrointestinal tract. Rich in menthol, peppermint eases stomach-aches, cramping, indigestion, nausea and vomiting, and addresses gall bladder dysfunction. Like many mints, it is also incredibly rich in volatile oils, making it a fitting remedy for colds, influenza, sinus infections and nasal congestion. The antibacterial, antimicrobial actions of the plant reduce problematic germs and aid the body to clear viral, bacterial and fungal infections, while the diaphoretic (sweat-inducing) properties assist by aiding the immune system in a protective manner. Topically, peppermint is a wonderful plant for skin irritations as it acts as an analgesic, reducing any associated pain.

The epitome of refreshment, even taking a deep inhale of peppermint will calm the nervous system and uplift the spirit.

PARTS USED

Leaves

ENERGETICS

Calming, cooling, spicy, drying, stimulating, relieving

ACTIONS

Antibacterial, antiemetic, antiseptic (gastrointestinal tract), antispasmodic (muscles), antitussive, aromatic, carminative, cholagogue, choleretic, cooling, diaphoretic, spasmolytic

CAUTIONS

Avoid during pregnancy and lactation as it may reduce milk flow. Caution in those with oesophageal reflux (especially the oil) and gallstones.

Plants for the People

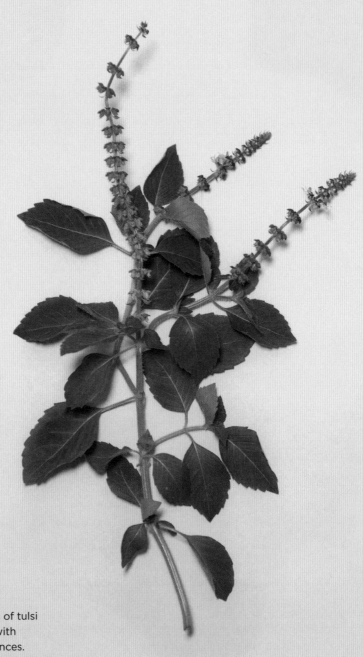

GOLDEN TIP

There are multiple types of tulsi
used medicinally, each with
slightly varying appearances.
In Ayurveda, they are called
Rama (green-leaved tulsi), Vana
(wild tulsi) and Krishna (purple-
leaved tulsi), to name a few.

OCIMUM TENUIFLORUM (SYN. OCIMUM SANCTUM)
TULSI

Dubbed the queen of herbs and also known as holy basil, tulsi has a bounty of regal common names, and rightly so. In Hinduism, it is revered as the embodiment of the goddess Tulsi, a sacred earthly manifestation of the goddess Lakshmi, and is said to bring blessings, good fortune and longevity. There is an esoteric aspect to tulsi that is said to harmonise the subtle energetic anatomies (chakras, meridians) of the body, mind and spirit.

Tulsi ignites the senses and is the most aromatic, delightful plant to grow; it honestly smells so good that the instinct is to get as close to it as humanly possible! When it flowers, the delicate blossoms stand tall along the lean stalks, and there is a resilience in the delicacy that speaks to the true nature of the plant. Tulsi is an adaptogenic tonic herb, essentially an anti-stress remedy with the ability to balance stress hormones (such as cortisol) in our bodies. It also acts positively on the nervous system to untangle and restore. Tulsi is wonderful for plumping up stamina and endurance, and to repair the vitality within that may be depleted from chronic exposure to stress. It has an impact on multiple systems in the body, from aiding detoxification of the liver to balancing blood sugar levels, providing cancer support, boosting immunity and harmonising digestion.

You can grow tulsi in the garden much like any common basil. In warmer climates, pick aplenty in bloom season as this will assist the plant to flourish in all its glory, so you can soak up 'the elixir of life' (another alias for tulsi!).

PARTS USED

Flowers, leaves, stalks, seeds, roots

ENERGETICS

Sweet, warming, heart opener, nourisher of the spirit

ACTIONS

Adaptogenic, alterative, antibacterial, antidepressant, antifungal, anti-inflammatory, antimicrobial, antioxidant, antiviral, anxiolytic, cardiotonic, carminative, demulcent, diaphoretic, expectorant, hepatoprotective, immunomodulator, nervine, radioprotective

CAUTIONS

Best to avoid during pregnancy and lactation, and when trying to conceive. Otherwise, it is very safe.

Plants for the People

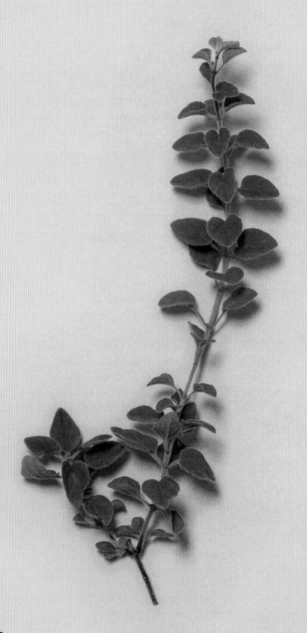

GOLDEN TIP

The whole oregano leaf is
perfect to add to steam
inhalations to shake congestion.

ORIGANUM VULGARE
OREGANO

Oregano, oh sweet oregano. Often overlooked beyond the spice rack, this is one marvellous healing plant we ought not disregard! The petite flowers and soft leaves are used for a wide array of conditions and have a strong tradition of medicinal use. Oregano is said to be ruled by the planet Venus, and Venus herself, the legendary Roman goddess of love, was thought to have grown and adored her oregano on Mount Olympus, creating the plant to bring happiness and joy.

Personally, I go straight to immunity and the gut when I connect to the medicine of oregano. It is a staple herb grown in our garden, often harvested when our household has been hit with the low-immunity stick. Oregano throws out a supercharged defence against viral or bacterial bugs, with strong antibacterial and antimicrobial actions that ease colds, influenza, fevers and upper respiratory tract infections. Oil of oregano is commonly used to treat fungal infections of all sorts topically and internally, and is generally renowned for combating digestive yeast (such as candida) and parasitic overgrowths. Oregano is also indicated for sluggish menstruation, indigestion, peptic ulceration and digestive weakness.

Overall, there is a calm, clearing and strengthening energy to this wonderful plant.

PARTS USED

Leaves, flowers

ENERGETICS

Warm, spicy, pungent, drying, stimulating, protective

ACTIONS

Anthelmintic, antibacterial, antifungal, antimicrobial, antioxidant, antiparasitic, antiseptic, carminative, expectorant, hypoglycaemic, stomachic

CAUTIONS

This is one strong plant, especially oil of oregano. The tiniest of quantities packs a punch, so be careful with dosing the oil. Take it encapsulated to maximise the effect on gut flora and to avoid burning the mucous membranes. If using the oil topically, dilute it with a neutral carrier oil, such as olive or almond.

Plants for the People

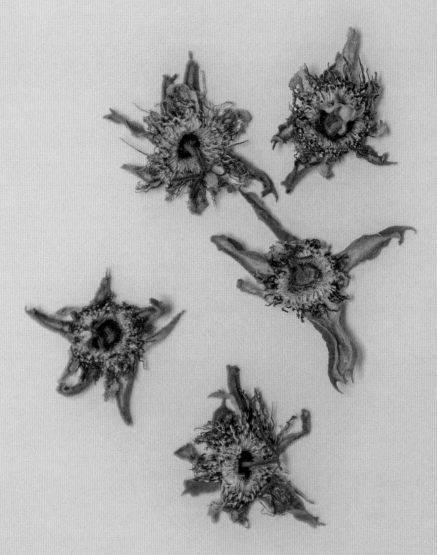

<u>GOLDEN TIP</u>

Passionflower amplifies its
medicine beautifully in combination
with other calming herbs, such
as valerian and chamomile.
Synergistically, they can relax
and settle the nervous system.

PASSIFLORA INCARNATA
PASSIONFLOWER

A tropical, creeping vine with a captivating, intricate flower. One of many species in the passionflower genus, *Passiflora incarnata* is well documented for its medicinal actions. From the Aztecs to the Native Americans, it has long been held in high regard for its healing strengths. In modern herbalism, the aerial parts of the plant are utilised, focusing on the flowers and leaves. Historically, the root has also been employed, although it is much less common nowadays to do so.

Passionflower has a delicate nature about it; we translate this as a remedy perfect for fragile folk, the young and the elderly. Kindred to the nervous system, passionflower works its magic for chronic insomnia and sleep issues, anxiety, restlessness, heart palpitations, irritability, headaches, muscle spasms, neuralgia, nervous tension, Parkinson's disease, seizures, and digestive upsets originating from a stressy belly. This is the epitome of a relaxing plant.

The sedative nature of passionflower makes it one of the mainstays in Western herbal medicine for all forms of sleep disorders. Passionflower's beautiful force eases the busy brain that may block our ability to claim deep rest; it will also kindly leave you without any lingering drowsiness in the morning. If you are experiencing a racing mind, anxiety or sleeplessness, call on this remedy. It will be of service with its inherently soothing song.

PARTS USED

Flowers, leaves

ENERGETICS

Cooling, drying, calming, softening, settling

ACTIONS

Anodyne, antispasmodic, anxiolytic, hypnotic, nervine, sedative

CAUTIONS

Generally a very safe plant, although not to be used during pregnancy. Exercise caution with pharmaceutical medications, especially monoamine oxidase inhibitors (MAOIs).

Plants for the People

165

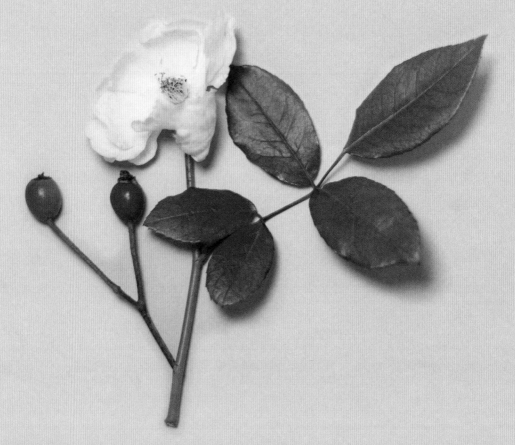

GOLDEN TIP

Rosehip powder is a delicious
addition to smoothies. The
powder is a freeze-dried form
of the fruit that maintains
all the medicinal bounty in a
much more accessible form.

ROSA CANINA
ROSEHIPS

Deep-ruby jewels emerging from forest-green foliage in the autumnal months, rosehips are most commonly harvested from the beautiful dog rose, *Rosa canina*, often found growing wild and free. Native Americans wove rosehips into their medicinal repertoire, as did Europeans in the World War II era, when the hips warded off scurvy with their supercharged vitamin C content.

The fresh raw fruit offers a world of antioxidant goodness. Abundant bioflavonoids and vitamin C enhance immunity and address a vitamin C deficiency, blurring the line between food and medicine beautifully. Rosehips address the underlying stressors that often contribute to lowered immune defence; they usher in warmth and are completely delightful for sore throats, colds and flu.

The heart responds well to rosehips – unsurprisingly, as the rose holds strong medicine akin to the heart. The antioxidants within the rosehips support the cardiovascular system and work overall to reduce systemic chronic inflammation, so they are great for varicose veins and all sorts of venous insufficiency. The hips are gently astringent, helpful in cases of diarrhoea and acting to cool overheated states of the body. Rosehips are often prescribed for arthritic conditions to prevent further degeneration and offer relief from joint pain, stiffness and aches. The sweet-and-sour fruits also show promising anti-ageing and anticancer effects. A floral superfood, fresh rosehips make the most excellent medicinal jam, fortifying immunity through the winter months.

PARTS USED

Whole fruits

ENERGETICS

Sour, warming, sweet

ACTIONS

Anti-inflammatory, antioxidant, antiscorbutic, astringent, diuretic, nutritive, stomachic

CAUTIONS

Caution with use during pregnancy and lactation, and by those with diabetic conditions or blood-related diseases.

Plants for the People

167

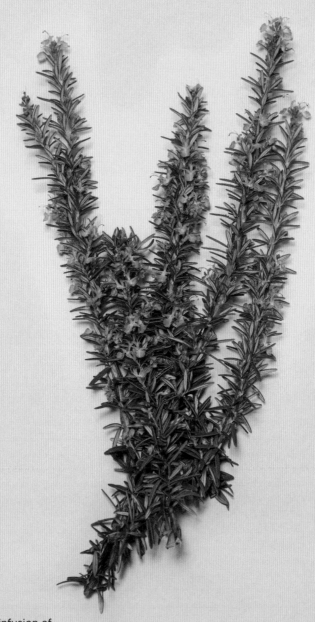

GOLDEN TIP

An olive oil–based infusion of
rosemary leaf massaged into
the scalp daily will stimulate
hair growth and encourage
luscious locks!

ROSMARINUS OFFICINALIS
ROSEMARY

Native to the Mediterranean, this ancient beauty has found its way into hearts and homes worldwide. Predominantly thought of as a culinary herb, and understandably so, rosemary creates an aromatic melody, igniting our senses as we chop and season with its greenery.

Medicinally, much of the historical use mirrors our current use. One stand-out application from the past that is still entirely relevant is as a powerful brain tonic, enhancing memory and sharpening concentration. The ancient Greeks held rosemary in high regard for this purpose alone. Nowadays, we value the great rosemary as a cerebral antioxidant for challenging neurological conditions such as ADHD, Parkinson's disease and Alzheimer's disease.

Super high in antioxidants, rosemary defends against free radicals with vigour. It soothes the nervous system, relieving tension headaches, easing anxiety and lifting depression, and encourages recovery from illness (especially if stress is at the root of the illness). Beyond these applications, rosemary is a key remedy for the cardiovascular system, improving poor circulation, reducing high blood pressure and aiding varicose veins; it oxygenates the blood and acts as a preventative akin to the heart. A plant with boundless indications, rosemary eases a gassy belly, stimulates appetite, cleanses, tonifies and protects the liver, slows the ageing process and assists the respiratory system when you are overcoming a cold or flu.

This fragrant evergreen has an uplifting essence and is well equipped and willing to stand tall by our sides with its pure, peaceful spirit.

PARTS USED

Leaves

ENERGETICS

Warming, drying, strengthening, stimulating, protective, unshakeable

ACTIONS

Analgesic (mild), antimicrobial, antioxidant, antispasmodic, carminative, cholagogue, circulatory stimulant, cognition enhancer, diuretic, hepatoprotective, hypotensive, nervine, rubefacient

CAUTIONS

Avoid during pregnancy.

Plants for the People

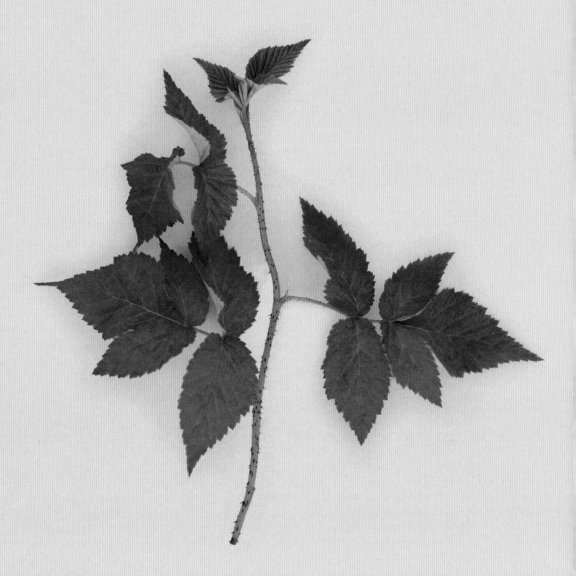

GOLDEN TIP

As raspberry leaf is tannin rich,
be sure to mix it up with other
herbs to avoid an overly drying
effect, especially if using it
long-term. A mix of raspberry
leaf and oat straw is a heavenly
balancing combination.

RUBUS IDAEUS
RASPBERRY LEAF

Red raspberry leaf is a uterus-centric herb, holding a deep connection with the female reproductive system. Throughout history, raspberry leaf tea has been drunk by expectant mothers as a partus preparator to relax and stimulate the womb for birth, prevent miscarriage and reduce the risk of birth complications.

These days, the nutritious leaf continues to be a powerful herbal assistant employed to encourage a healthy pregnancy and birth and a smooth post-birth recovery. It is said to aid restoration of the womb after birth, reducing the risk of haemorrhage while enhancing the richness of breastmilk – offering well-deserved assistance not only to the mamma but the babe too. The leaf can also be taken to calm nausea during pregnancy. However, it is not limited to pregnancy support; it is indicated to promote fertility, normalise menstrual imbalances and assist with premenstrual tension and irregular or painful, heavy periods. There is a strengthening and toning mechanism specific to the uterine and pelvic walls that enables raspberry leaf to send a wave of relief to the feminine forces.

I like to think of raspberry leaf as 'food as medicine', a natural multivitamin of sorts – it has a very high vitamin and mineral profile, making a superb nourishing tonic. Like the berries the plant produces, the leaf is packed full of vitamin C, alongside vitamins A, E and B, magnesium, potassium and calcium. Raspberry leaf tastes much like black tea, minus the caffeine, making it easy to drink daily. It has a high tannin profile (just as black tea does) and is wonderful for easing belly upsets, especially acute diarrhoea. The leaf is a perfect remedy for any inflammation of the mouth and throat, such as stomatitis or tonsillitis, and when applied topically is an effective antidote to conjunctivitis due to its astringent properties.

Energetically, raspberry leaf provides a very nutritive and cooling effect, just as it has for the wild women who came before us and will for the wild women who follow us.

PARTS USED

Leaves

ENERGETICS

Grounded, bitter, soothing, cooling

ACTIONS

Alterative (mild), antidiarrhoeal, antispasmodic, astringent, galactagogue, partus preparator, parturifacient, smooth muscle stimulant, uterine tonic

CAUTIONS

As evidence-based trials are not completely clear on when to begin taking raspberry leaf during pregnancy, this decision is often based on personal opinion and traditional use. Many believe it is safe to take throughout the whole pregnancy, but you will commonly see cautions to avoid it in the first trimester due to potential uterine stimulation, and advice to begin taking it in the more robust second and third trimesters. That said, it is noted both historically and currently to prevent miscarriage.

Steer clear in cases of constipation, malnutrition and iron-deficiency anaemia, due to the high tannins.

Plants for the People

171

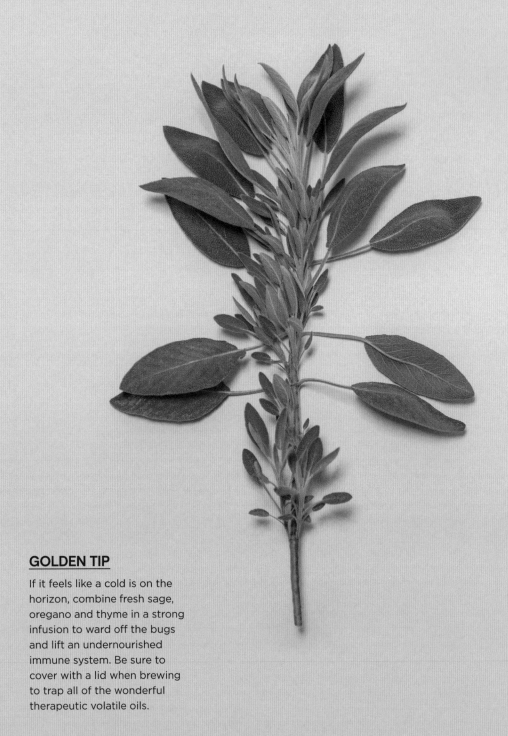

GOLDEN TIP

If it feels like a cold is on the
horizon, combine fresh sage,
oregano and thyme in a strong
infusion to ward off the bugs
and lift an undernourished
immune system. Be sure to
cover with a lid when brewing
to trap all of the wonderful
therapeutic volatile oils.

SALVIA OFFICINALIS
SAGE

This long-loved evergreen subshrub indigenous to the Mediterranean region is another culinary star with major medicinal abilities. Its name deriving from the Latin word *salvere*, meaning 'to be saved', sage is a wise, ancient force.

With strong antimicrobial abilities, sage defends inflamed mucous membranes and immunity, offering a tonic-like effect to fortify and protect against colds, fevers and flus. A simple infused throat gargle will bring much-needed relief and healing for canker sores, tonsillitis, pharyngitis, laryngitis, glossitis, stomatitis and gum disease. Sage has a hormone-balancing effect, promoting oestrogen flow, making it an ideal plant medicine for menopausal women, especially those battling night sweats and excessive heat.

One of the main indications for use is to decrease secretions, quietening overzealous saliva glands, inhibiting sweat, ceasing lactation, easing a runny nose, and calming excessive vaginal discharges and loose stools. A powerful aid for mammas who are experiencing an overflow of breastmilk, sage is certainly helpful when weaning infants. It is a fine plant for enhancing memory and concentration in conditions such as Alzheimer's disease and dementia. Sage also stimulates the liver and digestive system, aiding the breakdown of foods and cholesterol, reducing gas and indigestion.

PARTS USED

Leaves

ENERGETICS

Drying, pungent, cooling, bitter, relaxing, wise

ACTIONS

Antibacterial, antifungal, antigalactagogue, anhidrotic, antimicrobial, antioxidant, antiseptic (respiratory, gastrointestinal tract), antispasmodic, antiviral, aromatic, astringent, carminative

CAUTIONS

Avoid use during pregnancy! Please also avoid during lactation, unless wanting to decrease and cease milk supply.

Contains thujone, which in large amounts can be toxic. Although sage is relatively low in thujone, it is advised not to use high medicinal doses for extended periods of time – best to adhere to the daily recommended doses.

Plants for the People

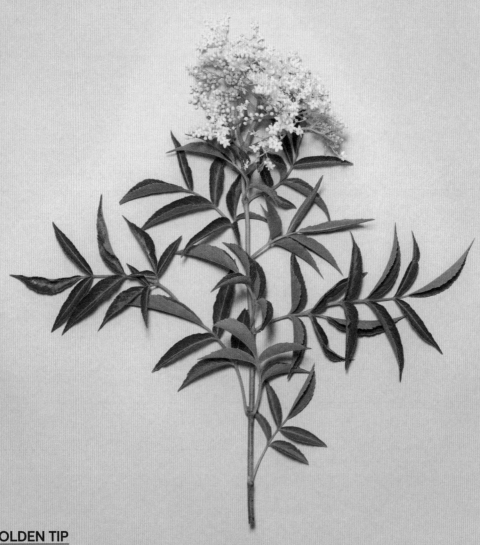

GOLDEN TIP

Cooked elderberries are a
delicious addition to the culinary
repertoire: the syrup imparts a
wonderful flavour when added
to kombucha brews or simmered
into tart jams. Also, the flowers
are the most beautiful edible
decoration.

SAMBUCUS NIGRA, SAMBUCUS CANADENSIS
ELDERBERRY/ELDERFLOWER

This wise old tree or shrub has umbrella-like, creamy-white flower heads and dark-purple, petite berry clusters that ripen over summer. Long revered in Europe, elder is a staple in most medicine cabinets to this day. It is wrapped in magical folklore, from ancient Roman to Celtic to Native American. *Sambucus nigra* is the European elder. There are quite a few types of elderberry that are very similar, such as the American elder, *Sambucus canadensis*.

Historically, the sacred elder tree's medicine was employed as a spring tonic, taken when the winter had passed and left its mark, with weary immune systems all round. Elderberry and elderflower are kindred to the immune system; both parts of the plant bring potent immune support with antiviral action. Ripe elderberries are commonly cooked down and made into a syrup, and I can safely say that this is one of the best tasting herbal remedies. Children (and adults) love this berry-rich, sweet elixir. The berries and flowers are used for upper respiratory congestion, coughs, colds, flu and sinusitis. The flowers are used to reduce fevers; they can bring on an active sweat to assist with breaking a fever while simultaneously stimulating the immune system to fight off any bugs or viruses. The flowers also have a strong cleansing effect, and the leaves are known for their topical benefits for bruising and wound relief.

PARTS USED

Berries and flowers, less commonly leaves and bark

ENERGETICS

Drying, cooling, fruitful, clearing, restorative

ACTIONS

Alterative (flowers, berries), anticatarrhal (flowers, berries), anti-inflammatory (flowers, berries), antioxidant (berries), antirheumatic (flowers, berries), antispasmodic (flowers, berries), antiviral (flowers, berries), aperient (flowers, berries), depurative (berries), diaphoretic (flowers), expectorant (flowers, berries), febrifuge (flowers), immunosupportive (flowers, berries), nervine (berries), vulnerary (berries, leaves)

CAUTIONS

Avoid eating the raw berries as they can bring on digestive discomfort if too many are ingested.

Not all elderberries are edible. Please identify your plant with accuracy when out wildcrafting!

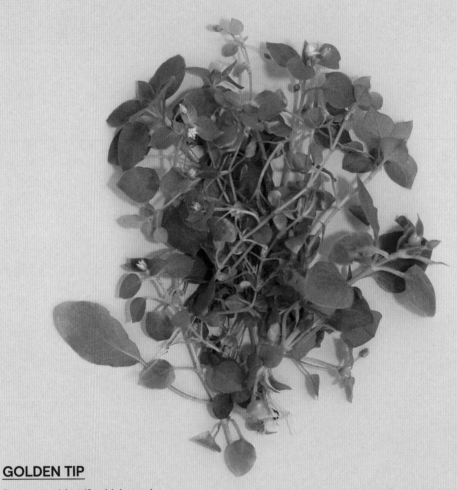

GOLDEN TIP

Be sure to identify chickweed
correctly. Once you do, you
can add it to a green salad,
juice the aerial parts, or cook it
up like spinach. Rich in amino
acids, B vitamins, vitamin C and
essential fatty acids, this is a
superb edible wild weed that
can be foraged daily.

WILD
WEED

STELLARIA MEDIA
CHICKWEED

Chickweed is a nutritious, edible, sprawling wild weed with delicate star-shaped, five-petalled white flower heads. One of our most common medicinal plants, it is superabundant, growing effortlessly worldwide in gardens, fields and wastelands, on sidewalks and along roadsides. The seeds of chickweed are said to germinate for up to sixty years – this is a persistent plant full of might and purpose.

Chickweed is incredibly valuable for topical use, predominantly in ointments, oils, balms, creams and poultices, bringing healing and tissue regeneration to the mucous membranes. An outstanding lubricating, cooling, soothing anti-inflammatory, it is indicated for all sorts of skin irritations. It counteracts dryness and itchiness, and is wonderful for eczema, psoriasis, dermatitis, bites, wounds, sunburn and rashes. In traditional Southern Appalachian folk medicine, chickweed eaten whole or taken in a tonic aids the assimilation of fats in digestion and balances lipid levels, even working to break up stones and cysts.

Taken orally, chickweed gently stimulates the lymphatic system, soothes the digestive system, and is perfect for use with gastrointestinal ulcerations to encourage repair and downgrade irritations. It is an epic counteractive plant medicine for a dry cough or dryness of the nasal passages, moistening and alleviating discomfort. This highly nourishing plant is a greatly underestimated healer – even using it as a rejuvenating daily tonic to green up your diet is massively beneficial.

PARTS USED

Flowers, leaves, stems

ENERGETICS

Cooling, soothing, moist, fresh, nourishing

ACTIONS

Anti-inflammatory, antipruritic, antiulcerogenic, astringent, demulcent, emollient, refrigerant, vulnerary

CAUTIONS

None known.

Plants for the People

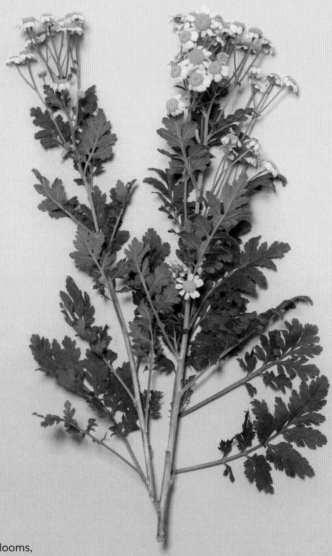

GOLDEN TIP

When a headache looms,
combine feverfew leaves and
flowers with lavender and lemon
balm to tame the tension. This
perfect trio unravels compressed
energy and switches off the
innate fight-or-flight response,
ushering in relief.

TANACETUM PARTHENIUM
FEVERFEW

The prettiest flowers spring from the buds of this medicinal plant in the warmer seasons. Often mistaken for chamomile, the blooms are a little more sturdy in energy and shape, clueing us in to the essence and actions of feverfew. Feverfew is the stand-out herbal remedy for migraines and associated symptoms such as nausea, dizziness and light sensitivity. In the modern apothecary, the herb is most commonly directed for prophylactic use over a long period of time for a marked relief in episodic migraines.

Feverfew has an uplifting nature, a sweet soothing energy, a lightness of being. It has long been a women's remedy; the ancient Greeks used it to stimulate delayed menses and as a birthing companion. An antiallergic plant with the ability to decrease histamine release, this is one stellar remedy for allergies, as well as for the common cold, flu and fever. Often prescribed for a variety of cramping, arthritic and skin conditions, feverfew harmonises the flow of blood, ushering in a cooling relief, much like a dip in a river on a warm summer's day, drawing out the overheated flames within.

PARTS USED

Leaves, flowers

ENERGETICS

Relieving, bitter, drying, cooling

ACTIONS

Analgesic, antiallergic, anti-inflammatory, antispasmodic, anthelmintic, bitter tonic, carminative, diaphoretic, emmenagogue, febrifuge, hepatoprotective, vasodilator

CAUTIONS

Avoid if sensitive to the Asteraceae (daisy) family, and during pregnancy and lactation. Caution in use with young children. In long-term use, mouth ulcerations and mucous membrane irritation has been noted as a side effect.

Plants for the People

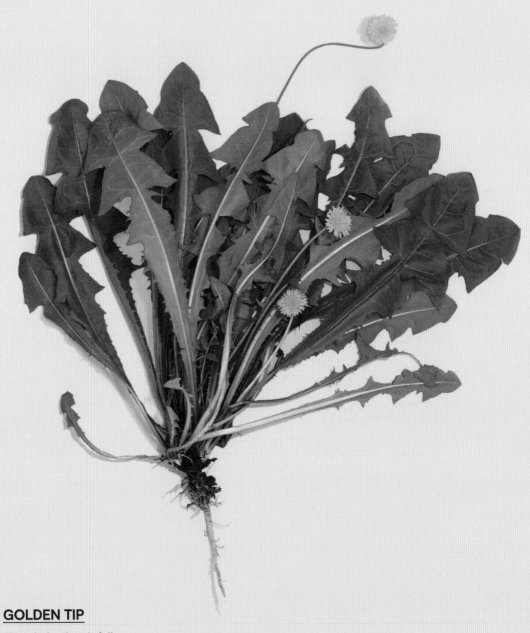

GOLDEN TIP

The whole plant is fully
edible – roots, flowers,
leaves, stem and buds.

TARAXACUM OFFICINALE
DANDELION

Abundant dandelion, full of might and perseverance, hails from the northern hemisphere. Come spring, this lawn-loving weed pops up, saluting the sun with its brilliant golden flower heads atop a lower circle of green, toothed leaves. When the plant goes to seed, a white halo-like globe replaces the flower. Dandelion grows anywhere and everywhere, a truly mineral-dense plant that replenishes depleted soils and depleted people. The roots reach deep into the earth, much like its medicine.

Dandelion has been used medicinally over the ages and across the continents, from the Romans, Persians and Native Americans to Eastern cultures. Moving stagnation and bringing cleansing, it is the ultimate spring tonic.

The roots are absolute liver-loving stars, working directly on liver congestion and promoting gall bladder health while supporting the connected emotions of these organs: anger, frustration, suppressed passions and rage. Dandelion is an effective detoxifier, digestive aid and blood cleanser with an underlying gentleness, which makes it a potent remedy for sluggish, sedentary, stressed systems. It is also high in potassium and vitamins A and C, which makes it incredibly restorative. The leaf acts as a formidable diuretic, wonderful for clearing fluid retention and bladder and kidney infections without further depleting the system, thanks to the mineral-rich elements contained within. The whole plant is incredibly useful – even the milky sap of the stem zaps warts, pimples and moles, and soothes insect bites when applied topically.

PARTS USED

Roots, flowers, leaves

ENERGETICS

Bitter, gentle, cooling, sweet, stimulating, drying, transformative

ACTIONS

Alterative (root), antirheumatic (leaf, root), aperient (root), bitter tonic (leaf, root), cholagogue (leaf, root), diuretic (leaf, root), laxative (leaf, root), stomachic (root)

CAUTIONS

Consult a healthcare practitioner if you have any existing gall bladder conditions; avoid if there are any bile duct or digestive obstructions present.

Plants for the People

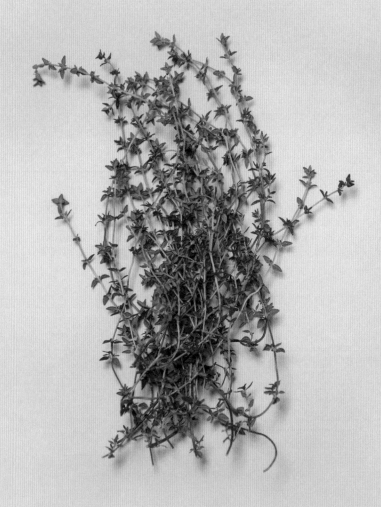

GOLDEN TIP

Rich in essential oil, thyme
is a perfect plant for use
in steam inhalations. The
aromatic aspects ignite
the senses and soothe the
symptoms of a common
cold and nasal congestion.

THYMUS VULGARIS
THYME

Although thyme has been used for eons, it is a vastly underestimated, undervalued plant ally in modern herbalism. Big mistake! Thyme is an incredible plant medicine with a rich history. Emperors were said to keep thyme close to protect them from poisoning, while ancient Romans and Greeks held it in high regard, giving it as a sign of respect and believing it brought energy, courage and bravery.

Thyme is a full-bodied herbal medicine with a penchant for immunity. It is wonderful for all sorts of upper respiratory congestion and inflammation, such as bronchial asthma, nasal catarrh, coughs, colds and influenza. With antimicrobial and antibacterial properties, thyme makes a gutsy germ-busting mouthwash for halitosis, dental decay, oral thrush, sore throats, tonsillitis and gingivitis. As kin to the thymus gland, it shakes up coughs and rigid mucus in a gentle way via its immune-enhancing mechanisms and relaxing expectorant action. Thyme also exerts a solid impact on the digestive system, easing excessive burping, bloating, diarrhoea, colic and belly spasms. Due to its strong disinfectant elements, thyme shines in topical use for acne, wounds, insect bites, stings, fungal overgrowths and so much more.

Full of hearty energy, this wonderful, invigorating herbal remedy deserves to claim a spot in your home apothecary for everyday support.

PARTS USED

Leaves, flowers

ENERGETICS

Vital, clearing, spicy, warming, drying

ACTIONS

Antibacterial, antifungal, antimicrobial, antioxidant, antiseptic (gastrointestinal tract), antispasmodic (respiratory tract), antitussive, antiviral, astringent, bronchodilator, carminative, digestive, expectorant, immune stimulant, rubefacient

CAUTIONS

Caution with use during pregnancy, otherwise thyme is a super-safe herb.

Plants for the People

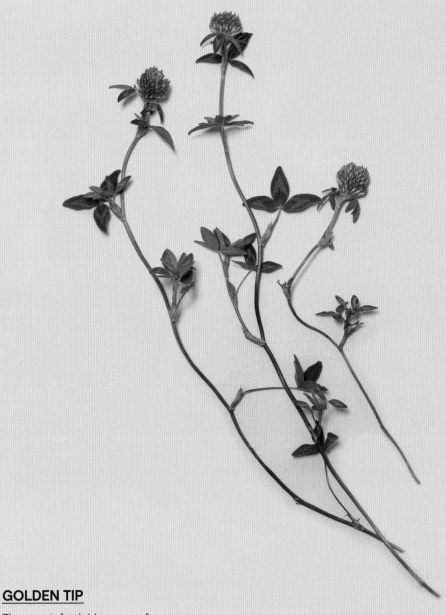

GOLDEN TIP

The sweet, fresh blossoms of
red clover taste delicious raw
and can be added to salads.

WILD WEED

TRIFOLIUM PRATENSE
RED CLOVER

Red clover has long held mystical powers. From protecting the Druids against the dark forces to its association with the triad goddesses among the ancient Romans and Greeks, the magic within the clover family is strong. Beloved by bees, the deep-pink young blossoms are a beautiful sight topping the lean, green stems and leaflets. Commonly found in lawns, fields, farmland and disturbed areas, red clover's flower head is the prime medicinal part of the plant used in Western herbal medicine.

Red clover is incredibly nutritious, containing a mineral-rich cocktail of iron, calcium, copper, magnesium, manganese and selenium, and an array of B vitamins and vitamin C, beta-carotene, bioflavonoids, isoflavones and inositol. It is a fantastic rebuilder and detoxifier, a most fitting herb for colds, coughs and bronchitis, indicated to clear respiratory complaints and shake up deep-set congestion. This pretty plant impacts the skin positively, clearing lymphatic congestion and chronic skin presentations, wonderful for acne, eczema, psoriasis and dermatitis. Historically used to treat cancers, today there is still a solid place for red clover in prevention and active cancer protocols. Red clover contains isoflavones (a type of phytoestrogen), which exert an oestrogenic effect on the body, calming menopausal symptoms such as hot flushes, night sweats and mood swings.

PARTS USED

Flowers, less commonly leaves

ENERGETICS

Cooling, sweet, salty, yin, clearing

ACTIONS

Alterative, anticancer, antispasmodic, depurative, expectorant, lymphatic, nutritive, oestrogenic

CAUTIONS

Recommended to avoid during pregnancy (although this is debated in the herbalist community).

Be cautious with oestrogen-dominant conditions such as endometriosis and uterine fibroids, or hormone-sensitive cancers (again, conflicting evidence and opinions exist).

Caution with use in haemophilia and by those prone to heavy bleeding; also avoid using concurrently with blood-thinning medications.

Plants for the People

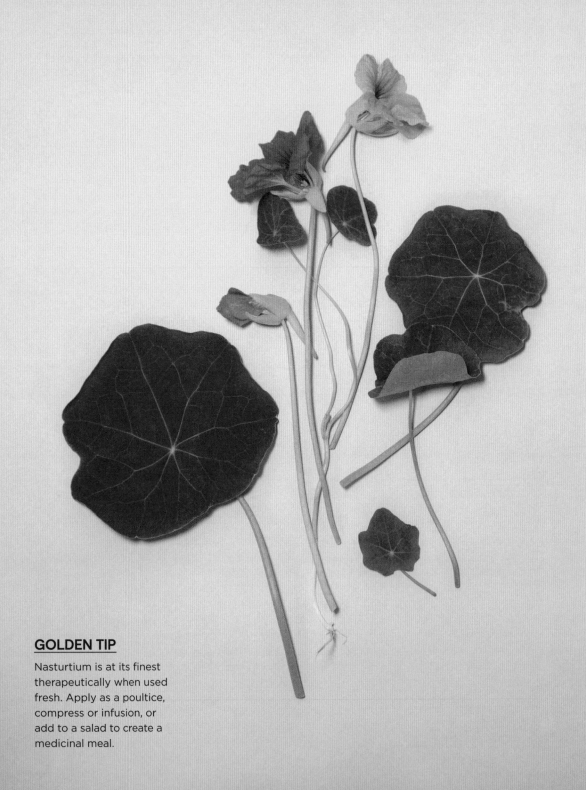

GOLDEN TIP

Nasturtium is at its finest
therapeutically when used
fresh. Apply as a poultice,
compress or infusion, or
add to a salad to create a
medicinal meal.

WILD
WEED

TROPAEOLUM MAJUS
NASTURTIUM

One of the most captivating flowers around, the nasturtium creates soft sprawling beauty wherever it plants itself. Bold orange, deep red and brilliant gold all pop profusely when the blooms begin. A relative of watercress, this is an edible plant, from the seed and leaf to the flower, wonderful in salads to add a peppery, crisp bite. The seeds are dubbed 'poor man's capers' and make a great substitute for the culinary caper. Nasturtium grows far from home; indigenous to the Andean region in South America, it has cast its seed worldwide and is now naturalised in many continents. As echoed throughout these pages, often the most fitting remedy is right by your side, and this self-seeding wonder weed is no exception.

Therapeutically, nasturtium possesses natural antibiotic properties and is effective on the respiratory and urinary systems. Nasturtium rises to offer its vitamin C–laden healing forces with cheer and willingness. It is a fitting choice to ward off the common cold, and wonderful for breaking up infections of all sorts, including bacterial infections. The seeds are naturally antifungal, while the leaves, stems and flowers contain more soothing elements that help treat infections of the upper respiratory tract and urinary tract. Overall, there is a strong combative support within the plant. Topically, nasturtium is a star for fungal infections and will also disinfect a cut or wound. The theme running through the whole plant is one of protection and harmony, inviting us to share the strengths that exist in the folds of such beauty.

PARTS USED

Leaves, seeds, flowers

ENERGETICS

Spicy, pungent, warming, uplifting

ACTIONS

Antibacterial, antibiotic, antifungal, cholagogue, disinfectant, diuretic, expectorant

CAUTIONS

Caution with use during pregnancy and lactation.

Plants for the People

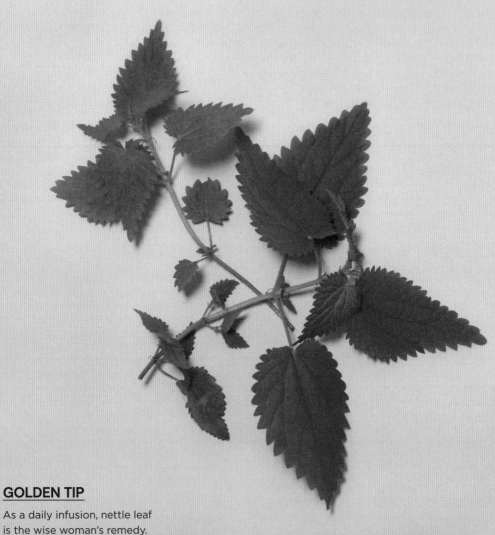

GOLDEN TIP

As a daily infusion, nettle leaf
is the wise woman's remedy.
The rich deep-green leaves
create a tonic full of might.
For sensitive folk, nettle is
best anchored with a calming,
grounded companion such
as oat straw.

WILD
WEED

URTICA DIOICA
NETTLE

The story of nettle is as rich as the leaf is green. Nettle is an ever-present plant in our history; once commonly used for textiles, this wild weed has myriad applications and a definite mystical presence. In many traditions, the plant was kept close to ward off bad vibes and protect from the dark forces. Also known as stinging nettle, the plant does just as the name suggests, which demands the forager be mindful when working with it to avoid a formic acid–rich sting. Thankfully, the sting is neutralised by cooking or drying, making the edible, nutrient-dense leaves perfect to blanch for pesto and to add to soups. A powerful blood-building tonic, nettle leaf is packed with iron, calcium, potassium, zinc, magnesium, silica, fibre, protein, chlorophyll, B vitamins, vitamin A and vitamin C.

Nettle's most famed folk use is 'urtication' – essentially flogging bare skin with the stinging plant to provoke inflammation to ease rheumatic pains, which reportedly can provide up to a week of relief. These days we value nettle for much gentler applications.

There are three parts used medicinally: the leaves predominantly, and less commonly the seeds and roots. These are almost like three entirely individual medicines; they each have such varied applications. The seed is nutrient dense and used to combat fatigue, while the root is mainly used for prostate issues and urinary tract infections. All parts of the plant, in fact, aid the kidneys and the urinary system. The leaf is heavily indicated for arthritis, osteoarthritis, rheumatic pain and liver health alongside inflammatory skin conditions, such as eczema, dermatitis and urticaria. The leaf works to nourish the body on a cellular level, supporting connective tissue repair and replenishing deficiencies. As nettle leaf tones the tissues within, it can be applied to many organ systems, from the uterus to the intestines.

Nettle is a plant that is exceptionally hard to summarise as it is useful in so many scenarios. Primarily, connect with nettle for its nourishment – it is the most fitting remedy for those struggling with anaemia and nutrient depletion – and for its in-built wisdom, raising the vital forces within and removing stagnation.

Plants for the People

PARTS USED

Leaves, seeds, roots

ENERGETICS

Drying, cooling, stimulating, reconnecting, wholesome, clearing

ACTIONS

Alterative, antihistamine, anti-inflammatory, antiprostatic (root), astringent, circulatory stimulant, diuretic, galactagogue, haemostatic, hypoglycaemic, nutritive, trophorestorative, styptic

CAUTIONS

Always wear gloves when foraging nettles as they pack a mighty sting! Caution with use during pregnancy and lactation.

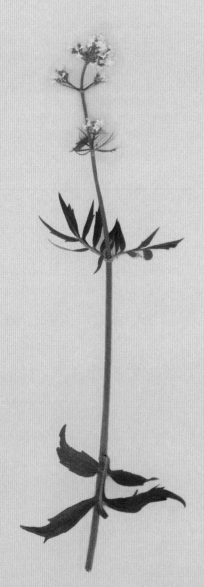

GOLDEN TIP

Do not dismiss the efficacy
of valerian if you do not feel an
instant effect after one dose.
This plant medicine is best used
for a solid 1–2 weeks to really
sink in and work its magic.

VALERIANA OFFICINALIS
VALERIAN

Some of you will be lucky enough to live in an environment where valerian is deemed a wild weed. The creamy-white to blush-pink flowers are a beautiful sight on the impressively upright, vigorous plant. Valerian is known for its distinctive smell – there really is nothing quite like it! An ally for the nervous system, even the Latin name encompasses the plant's spirit, *valere* meaning 'to be strong, be well'. Hippocrates and Dioscorides recorded the use of valerian as a sleep aid, and during World War II it was used to calm people's nerves as they lived through this frightening time.

Valerian aims to part the stormy clouds and let the light shine in, quietening frenetic energy to ease anxiety and panic attacks, calm a busy, irritable mind and hum a lullaby for those battling insomnia and sleepless nights. This powerful root is indicated for restlessness in all forms, including cramps, muscular spasms and pains. Most commonly thought of for its sedative powers, valerian is not limited to these by any means. It eases hypertension, aids menstrual flow, and relieves migraines, rheumatic complaints and intestinal colic. This plant medicine reminds us that although our reactions to stressful situations are completely valid, we can always find our way back to our centre.

PARTS USED

Roots, rhizome

ENERGETICS

Warming, relaxing, moving, clears burdens and excess stimuli, light-bringing

ACTIONS

Antispasmodic (muscles), anxiolytic, carminative, hypnotic, hypotensive, nervine, sedative

CAUTIONS

Avoid use during pregnancy and lactation. Be mindful of dosing in the daytime, especially if needing to be at your sharpest or operating heavy machinery, as valerian has a marked sedative effect that may impair your senses.

Plants for the People

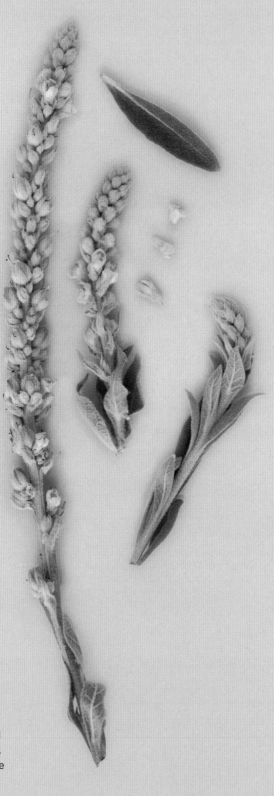

GOLDEN TIP

The sunny flowers of mullein
are used to make a soothing
distilled ear oil (especially in
combination with garlic oil),
and the leaves are best dried
for a respiratory-support tea.
The root is best utilised in the
form of a tincture.

WILD
WEED

VERBASCUM THAPSUS
MULLEIN

A striking weedy wonder with sulphur-yellow popping flowers along a tall stem growing up to 2 metres (6½ feet) high, and soft, furry, droopy leaves, this is a hard-to-miss plant in the wild, where it grows in all sorts of terrain. Happily common and wonderfully useful, mullein is old-world medicine, a much-loved folk remedy in European and Native American traditions, with applications ranging from hair dye to warding off evil forces and protecting against dark magic. On the lighter side, mullein was thought to fortify courage and love.

Mullein has been naturalised worldwide. It was introduced to Australia and North America with colonisation and is mistakenly thought to have originated in the soils of the Americas. Native Americans adopted the plant into their healing traditions, smoking the leaf, often to relieve asthma and bronchial congestion. Spanning many cultures and times, the leaves have been used for poultices to alleviate arthritic symptoms and aid healing of cuts and wounds.

Modern herbalism praises mullein for its affinity with the respiratory system. The leaf has a strong soothing action to ease an irritated dry cough and hoarseness, and acts as an expectorant to shake up lung congestion. It is a key plant indicated for allergies, asthma and all bronchial afflictions. Commonly utilised externally for earaches and ear infections, the flowers are used in an oil infusion to soften symptoms. Mullein root, on the other hand, has a strong rapport with the kidneys, bladder and gastrointestinal tract. It is a wonderful lymphatic stimulator and works to move through any glandular stagnation – think swollen glands, glandular fever, bites and stings, and bruising.

PARTS USED

Flowers, leaves, roots

ENERGETICS

Cooling, supportive, moistening

ACTIONS

Anodyne, antibacterial, anti-inflammatory, antiseptic, antitussive, astringent, demulcent, emollient, expectorant, lymphatic, nervine (mild), vulnerary

CAUTIONS

None known.

Plants for the People

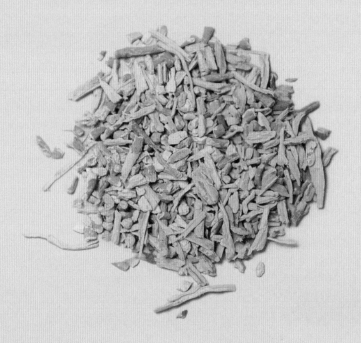

GOLDEN TIP

Create an anupan, a traditional
Ayurvedic medicine by combining
fine-powdered ashwagandha
root with golden ghee and raw
honey for a delicious daily dose
to strengthen and fortify.

WITHANIA SOMNIFERA
ASHWAGANDHA

A favoured root of our times, ashwagandha is in vogue these days, which makes a whole lot of sense when we understand its powers. A consistently revered Ayurvedic tonic recorded in the Sanskrit sacred texts, ashwagandha is also lovingly dubbed the Indian ginseng. The common name roughly translates to 'the strength of a horse', alluding to the deeper strengths within. This plant is a supreme being, a restorer of the young and old, a prime adaptogenic tonic. An adaptogen essentially holds anti-stress powers and has the ability to speak to our bodies to help them adapt to stressors and nourish the systems involved in responding. Cortisol, a key stress hormone, is regulated in a supportive manner by ashwagandha, aiding the often depleted adrenal glands. Not only is this key for our energy, vitality and nervous system, it is vital for our reproductive system. There is a libido-enhancing essence within the root, which could be due to the overall enhancing effect on longevity.

We employ ashwagandha for exhausted, undernourished, burnt-out, convalescing folk. For those struggling with chronic low energy, this plant medicine is heavily indicated, so call it in if you are experiencing chronic fatigue syndrome, fibromyalgia or post-viral symptoms that are hard to shake. Ashwagandha assists the cardiovascular system, immunity, sleep and endurance, and increases cognitive clarity and sharpness. It is a root for those who are empty and worn out. It is also a true friend for those weathering serious pathologies such as cancer, addictions, emaciation, HIV and AIDS, and neurodegenerative diseases. Essentially known as an antioxidant, the plant exerts an anticancer immune-stimulating effect and has proven to be a valued adjunct therapy for chemotherapy and radiation treatment. The leaves have a wound-healing impact and can be applied topically to ease cuts and inflammation. A most rejuvenative tonic!

PARTS USED

Primarily roots, occasionally leaves, rarely seeds and flowers

ENERGETICS

Warming, sweet, earthing, restorative

ACTIONS

Adaptogenic, alterative, anticancer, anti-inflammatory, antitumour, anxiolytic, hypotensive, nervine, neuroprotective, nootropic, sedative (mild), tonic

CAUTIONS

Not for use during pregnancy. Ashwagandha belongs to the Solanaceae (nightshade) family and in rare cases may be inflammatory for those with sensitivities to this group of plants.

Plants for the People

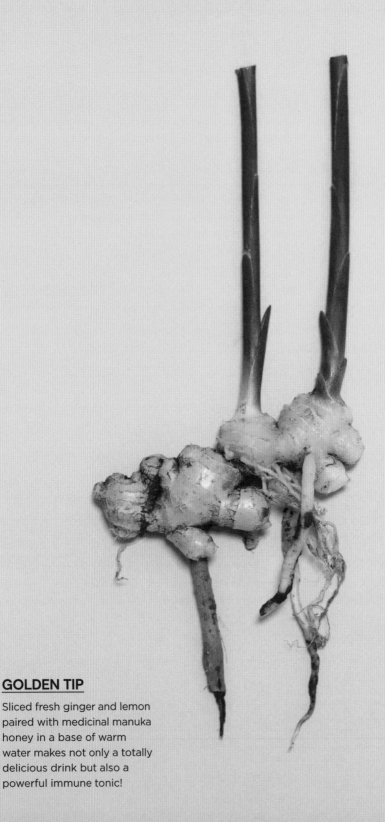

GOLDEN TIP

Sliced fresh ginger and lemon
paired with medicinal manuka
honey in a base of warm
water makes not only a totally
delicious drink but also a
powerful immune tonic!

ZINGIBER OFFICINALE
GINGER

Ginger warms like no other remedy. It is famed for igniting a flush of heat, and a time does not exist in the history of folk medicine when this versatile rhizome has not been in use from the East to the West. The ancient Indians dubbed ginger 'maha oushadha', the great medicine, and it is treasured in Ayurveda for its tonifying qualities and infinite uses. When Hippocrates spoke his famous words 'Let food be thy medicine, and medicine be thy food', perhaps he was referencing sweet and peppery ginger! A king in the kitchen, this antioxidant-rich super spice is loaded with medicinal potential.

Ginger acts as a warming stimulant on the respiratory system and is most commonly utilised to ward off a cold or sore throat, and for asthma, bronchial infections and congestion. It also has anti-nausea properties and so is indicated to relieve side effects during and after chemotherapy treatments, postoperative nausea, and morning, motion and sea sickness. Our guts simply adore ginger – this hero food addresses digestive weakness, relieving bloating, gas, colic and indigestion.

Incredible for colder constitutions, the heat of the rhizome encourages circulatory flow, which in addition to its marked antispasmodic, pain-relieving power can be very helpful for painful menstrual cramping and endometriosis. Ginger also holds the ability to repair and soothe a multitude of arthritic conditions and symptoms due to its mammoth anti-inflammatory profile and nourishing fire. It is known to balance chaotic blood sugar levels and lower elevated cholesterol – the therapeutic benefits of this rhizome are unending!

Ginger's medicine is invigorating – it is a lifting, boosting, shifting force, an entirely flexible antioxidant-rich cocktail glowing with warmth.

PARTS USED

Rhizome

ENERGETICS

Warming, drying, stimulating, awakening

ACTIONS

Analgesic, antiemetic, anti-inflammatory, antiplatelet, aromatic, cardioprotective, carminative, demulcent, diaphoretic, expectorant, metabolic stimulant, peripheral vasodilator, rubefacient, stimulant

CAUTIONS

Avoid high doses during pregnancy; steer clear if peptic ulcerations or gallstones are present. Use cautiously with extreme gastric sensitivities.

Plants for the People

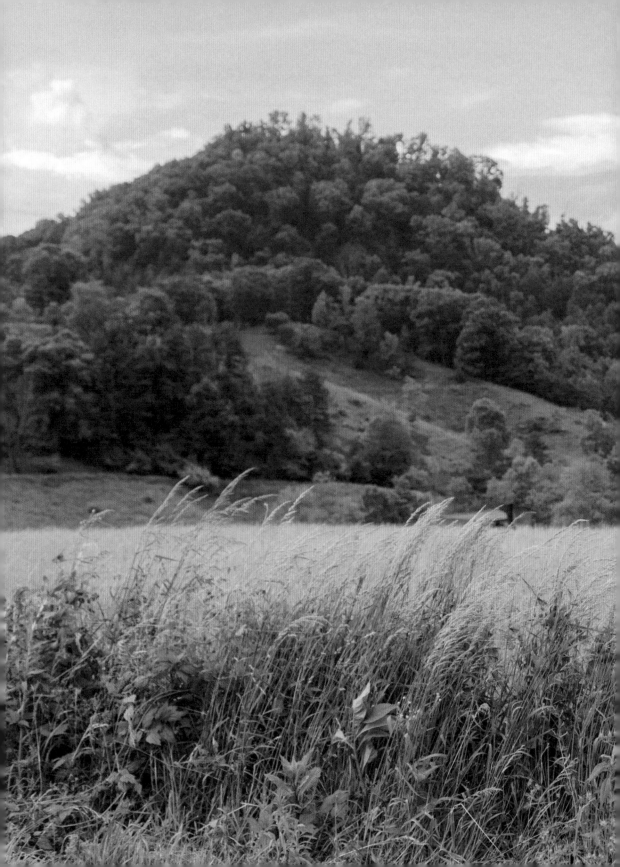

GLOSSARY

ADAPTOGENIC
Enhances the inner defences against the harmful impacts of stressors on the body; supports the ability to adapt to stress while promoting physiological functions.

ADRENAL MODULATOR
Normalises adrenal gland/hypothalamic-pituitary-adrenal (HPA) axis.

ALTERATIVE
Restores balance within the body, purifies and cleanses the blood, creates a metabolic tonic-like effect, raising vitality and wellbeing.

AMENORRHOEA
The absence of a menstrual cycle, generally three or more consecutive menstrual cycles.

ANALGESIC
Pain reliever when taken orally.

ANHIDROTIC
Reduces sweating.

ANODYNE
Pain reliever when applied externally.

ANTHELMINTIC
Targets intestinal worms.

ANTIALLERGIC
Calms allergy responses and reduces histamine release.

ANTIARRHYTHMIC
Normalises irregular heartbeats and rhythms.

ANTIATHEROSCLEROTIC
Counteracts the effects of atherosclerosis (plaque build-up within the arteries).

ANTIBACTERIAL
Destroys and defends against bacterial growths.

ANTIBIOTIC
Inhibits the growth of or destroys microorganisms.

ANTICANCER
Protects against and counteracts cancer growth and formation.

ANTICATARRHAL
Reduces mucus.

ANTICOAGULANT
Inhibits blood coagulation.

ANTICONVULSANT
Prevents and reduces seizures and convulsions.

ANTIDEPRESSANT
Alleviates depression.

ANTIDIABETIC
Alleviates diabetes and diabetic symptoms.

ANTIDIARRHOEAL
Relieves and prevents diarrhoea.

ANTIEMETIC
Relieves and reduces nausea and vomiting.

ANTIFIBROTIC
Defends against and prevents the growth of excess fibrous tissue.

ANTIFUNGAL
Defends against and inhibits fungal and yeast infections.

ANTIGALACTAGOGUE
Inhibits breastmilk production and flow.

ANTIHAEMORRHAGIC
Calms and stops internal bleeding.

ANTIHISTAMINE
Reduces histamine response, beneficial for allergies.

ANTIHYPERTENSIVE
Specific for hypertension; reduces blood pressure.

ANTI-INFLAMMATORY
Reduces and counteracts inflammation.

ANTILIPIDEMIC
Reduces blood lipid levels, often employed to lower cholesterol.

ANTIMALARIAL
Used to protect against malaria and alleviate associated symptoms.

ANTIMICROBIAL
Defends against and inhibits microbial growths.

ANTIOXIDANT
Protects cells and scavenges free radicals to inhibit oxidation.

ANTIPARASITIC
Defends against and eradicates parasites.

ANTIPLATELET
Lowers blood platelet aggregation and improves arterial circulation; reduces the risk of clotting.

ANTIPROSTATIC
Alleviates prostate symptoms.

ANTIPROTOZOAL
Eradicates and inhibits protozoal infections.

ANTIPRURITIC
Calms and relieves itching.

ANTIRHEUMATIC
Alleviates and reduces the symptoms of rheumatism.

ANTISCORBUTIC
Corrects and prevents scurvy; rich in vitamin C.

ANTISEPTIC
Prevents infection and eradicates harmful organisms.

ANTISPASMODIC
Eases spasms of all kinds.

ANTITHYROID
Suppresses thyroid functions.

ANTITUMOUR
Reduces and counteracts tumour growth.

ANTITUSSIVE
Suppresses the cough reflex.

ANTIULCEROGENIC
Prevents and heals ulcerations.

ANTIVIRAL
Inhibits viruses.

ANXIOLYTIC
Eases and reduces anxiety.

APERIENT
Relieves constipation, a mild laxative.

AROMATIC
A group of essential oil–rich plants that soothe digestive functions, relieving gas.

ASTRINGENT
Causes tissues and mucous membranes to contract.

ATHEROSCLEROSIS
The build-up of substances, such as fats and cholesterol, within the arteries, causing thickening and hardening of the arterial walls.

BITTER TONIC
Stimulates gastric juices via bitter taste, aiding appetite and digestion.

BRONCHODILATOR
Widens the bronchi for improved airflow into the lungs.

CARDIOPROTECTIVE
Protects the heart from poor function, damage, toxins, disease and injury.

CARDIOTONIC
Strengthens the cardiovascular system.

CARMINATIVE
Reduces flatulence, usually by relaxing intestinal sphincter muscles.

CHEMOPROTECTIVE
Protects against the toxins and side effects of anticancer treatments.

CHOLAGOGUE
Encourages and stimulates the flow of bile from the gall bladder.

CHOLERETIC
Increases the volume of bile produced by the liver.

CIRCULATORY STIMULANT
Enhances the circulation of blood.

COGNITION ENHANCER
Enhances mental sharpness, concentration and alertness.

COLLAGEN SYNTHESISER
Promotes collagen synthesis.

CONNECTIVE-TISSUE REGENERATOR
Assists the regeneration of tissues.

DEMULCENT
Relieves irritations via a soothing, protective, nurturing effect.

DEPURATIVE
Aids purification and detoxification of body systems.

DIAPHORETIC
Encourages sweating.

DIGESTIVE
Aids digestion.

DISINFECTANT
Destroys bacteria.

DIURETIC
Increases urination and encourages metabolic waste product excretion.

DYSMENORRHOEA
Painful menstrual cycle and/or cramping.

EMMENAGOGUE
Stimulates the uterus and supports menstrual flow.

EMOLLIENT
Protects, softens and soothes the skin.

EXPECTORANT
Encourages phlegm and mucus to shift from the throat and lungs.

FEBRIFUGE
Eases and actively reduces a fever.

GALACTAGOGUE
Assists the production and flow of breastmilk.

HAEMOSTATIC
Stops blood loss – the first stage of wound healing.

HEPATOPROTECTIVE
Protects the liver from damage.

HYDROSOL
An aromatic water made by steam distillation of floral parts, leaves, fruits and plant materials.

HYPNOTIC
Sedative and powerful nervine; induces sleep.

HYPOCHOLESTEROLEMIC
Lowers blood cholesterol levels.

HYPOGLYCAEMIC
Balances and regulates blood sugar levels.

HYPOTENSIVE
Lowers blood pressure.

IMMUNE ENHANCING
Positively impacts the immune system by boosting functions.

IMMUNOMODULATOR
Regulates and normalises the immune system.

IMMUNOSUPPORTIVE
Protects and enhances immune system functions.

LAXATIVE
Stimulates and facilitates bowel movement.

LYMPHATIC
Detoxifies and supports fluid flow within the lymphatic system, impacting blood cleansing and stagnancy.

METABOLIC STIMULANT
Stimulates the metabolism and basal metabolic rate.

MUCOLYTIC
Breaks down and thins mucus.

MUCOPROTECTIVE
Protects mucous membranes.

NERVINE
Relaxes, strengthens and calms the nervous system.

NEUROPROTECTIVE
Protects the nervous system against damage from injury and degeneration.

NEUROREGENERATIVE
Promotes repair and regeneration of the nervous system.

NOOTROPIC
Enhances cognitive functions, memory, creativity and motivation; facilitates learning.

NUTRITIVE
Nourishes; rich in vitamins and minerals.

OESTROGEN MODULATOR
Moderates oestrogen receptors and oestrogen activity in the body.

OESTROGENIC
Stimulates oestrogen receptor sites and pathways.

ONEIROGEN
Enhances consciousness and dream-like states.

OREXIGENIC
Encourages appetite.

PARTURIFACIENT
Aids birth by inducing and assisting labour, contractions and placenta delivery.

PARTUS PREPARATOR
Specific to the second and third trimester of pregnancy; prepares the body for labour and birthing.

PERIPHERAL VASODILATOR
Widens the peripheral blood vessels, promoting circulation and tissue health, thereby reducing blood pressure.

PURGATIVE
Causes the evacuation of the bowels; much stronger than a general laxative.

RADIOPROTECTIVE
Protects against the toxins and side effects of anticancer treatments and radiation exposure.

REFRIGERANT
Cools and lowers body temperature; relieves fever and thirst.

RELAXANT
Non-drowsy tension tamer; calms the body and eases pain.

RUBEFACIENT
Causes reddening of the skin and improved circulation when applied topically.

SEDATIVE
Promotes sleep by relaxing the nervous system; reduces excitability and nervousness.

SIALAGOGUE
Promotes the flow of saliva.

SMOOTH MUSCLE STIMULANT
Stimulates smooth (involuntary) muscle fibres, such as those in the colon.

STIMULANT
Quickens the activity of a body system or organ.

STOMACHIC
Strengthens and tones the stomach; increases appetite and aids digestion.

STYPTIC
Stops bleeding via vascular contraction.

THYMOLEPTIC
Raises moods and lifts the spirit with a natural antidepressant-like effect.

TONIC
Restorative for the whole system or a particular system/organ, encouraging health and vitality.

TROPHORESTORATIVE
Restores and nourishes a particular system or organ in the body.

TSH ANTAGONIST
Blocks thyroid stimulating hormone (TSH) activity.

UTERINE STIMULANT
Stimulates the uterus.

UTERINE TONIC
Tones and strengthens the uterus.

VASODILATOR
Widens blood vessels.

VULNERARY
Encourages wound healing.

RESOURCES

BOTANICAL MEDICINE MAKING SUPPLIERS

Australia

Dried herbs: organic, wildcrafted and conventional
australherbs.com.au

Certified organic, Australian-grown dried herbs
highlandherbs.com.au

Medicinal plants, dried herbs, herb seeds; herbal bookshop
allrareherbs.com.au

Medicinal plants, dried herbs, tea supplies, bottles and jars
herbcottage.com.au

Bottles and jars
plasdene.com.au

USA

Dried herbs, tea supplies, bottles and jars
mountainroseherbs.com
starwest-botanicals.com

Seasonal, fresh plant material; dried herbs and seeds
pacificbotanicals.com

Seasonal, fresh plant material
sonomaherbs.org

UK

Dried and fresh herbs
organicherbtrading.com

Dried herbs, tea supplies, bottles and jars
baldwins.co.uk

WILDCRAFTING GUIDES AND INSIGHTS

Botany in a Day: The Patterns Method of Plant Identification (6th ed.), Thomas J. Elpel, HOPS Press, 2013.

The Forager's Harvest: A Guide to Identifying, Harvesting, and Preparing Edible Wild Plants, Samuel Thayer, Forager's Harvest Press, 2006.

Foraging & Feasting: A Field Guide and Wild Food Cookbook (2nd ed.), Dina Falconi, Botanical Arts Press, 2013.

Identifying and Harvesting Edible and Medicinal Plants, Steve Brill and Evelyn Dean, William Morrow and Company, 2010 (first published 1994).

Nature's Garden: A Guide to Identifying, Harvesting, and Preparing Edible Wild Plants, Samuel Thayer, Forager's Harvest Press, 2010.

Newcomb's Wildflower Guide, Lawrence Newcomb, Little, Brown and Company, 1989.

Peterson Field Guide to Medicinal Plants and Herbs of Eastern and Central North America (3rd ed.), Steven Foster and James A. Duke, Houghton Mifflin Harcourt, 2014.

The Weed Forager's Handbook: A Guide to Edible and Medicinal Weeds in Australia, Adam Grubb and Annie Raser-Rowland, Hyland House Publishing, 2012.

PLANT CONSERVATION CRUSADERS

unitedplantsavers.org
sustainableherbsproject.com

CLASSIC TEXTS FOR FURTHER READING

The Book of Herbal Wisdom: Using Plants As Medicines, Matthew Wood, North Atlantic Books, 1997.

The Herbal Medicine-Maker's Handbook, James Green, Crossing Press, 2000.

Holistic Herbal: A Safe and Practical Guide to Making and Using Herbal Remedies (4th ed.), David Hoffman, Thorsons, 2003.

Making Plant Medicine, Richo Cech, Horizon Herbs, 2000.

Medical Herbalism: The Science and Practice of Herbal Medicine, David Hoffmann, Inner Traditions Bear and Company, 2003.

Planetary Herbology, Michael Tierra, Lotus Press, 1988.

Plant Spirit Healing: A Guide to Working with Plant Consciousness, Pam Montgomery, Inner Traditions Bear and Company, 2008.

Planting the Future: Saving Our Medicinal Herbs, Rosemary Gladstar and Pamela Hirsch (eds), Healing Arts Press, 2000.

Rosemary Gladstar's Herbal Recipes for Vibrant Health, Rosemary Gladstar, Storey Publishing, 2008.

Plants for the People

ACKNOWLEDGEMENTS

To all the teachers, guides, mentors and wise ones who paved the way for me to continue, I see you and thank you.

To my publisher, Kirsten Abbott. You have championed this book from day one, and I am endlessly grateful for your vision and belief in me. Deepest thanks to the Thames & Hudson team, and to all who helped bring this book to life.

To my dear friend, collaborator and photographer, Georgia Blackie. Thank you for your wonderful, straight-up magical talent. From the wilds of the Byron Bay hinterland in Australia to the coasts of California, the deep forests of Tennessee and the open fields of North Carolina, you connected with the plants every step of the way, talking to them, meeting the land. And in turn, everything seemed to awaken and dance for you to capture its beauty. I am endlessly thankful to you, Georgia.

To my wise herbalist sisters Sarah Mann, Lauren Haynes and Jacqui Bushell. Your feedback, encouragement and support meant the world to me while I was writing this book.

To all who contributed recipes – Sarah, Lauren, Kira, Justina – I thank you wholeheartedly. To be in a community with you is a very special thing.

Plants for the People gave me the opportunity to step onto slices of land abundant with heavenly herbals as many kind souls opened their gardens, farms and homes. Thanks to Manu and her bountiful garden; to the kindest Chrissy and Cindy; to Rebecca at the California School of Herbal Studies; to Karen of Petalland Flower and Herb Farm; to the incredible Lisa of Pipsissewa Herbs; to Joe Hollis of Mountain Gardens; to Katie and Mike of Lady Luck Flower Farm; to Gabe of Pangaea Plants; to Saralyn of Heilbron Herbs; and to the kind folk at Gaia Herbs. Visiting you fortified the heartbeat of herbalism for me. We are united in our roles as guardians of the plant wisdoms, and you all inspired me greatly. Thank you warmly.

To my Uncle Les, who is no longer with us on this earthly plane. I did not realise how much my childhood experience of gardening by your side shaped my connection to the plants until I sat down to write this book. So thank you, old chappy. I hope that wherever you are there is an endless supply of chestnuts and rock cakes – your favourites.

To my dear friends and family, who have cheered me on and offered me nothing but encouragement and strength to bring this book through, I love you.

For my sunshiners: my mum, Leah, and my dad, Peter. There are few words to express how much I love you both, and how much your belief in me and enduring support have shaped me so greatly. You are my heroes.

To my constant canine companions Clark, Quinn and Hank. There could be no better company than you three.

And finally, but mightily. For my husband, Noah. Thank you, thank you, thank you. Your unshakable presence in my life is simply everything to me.

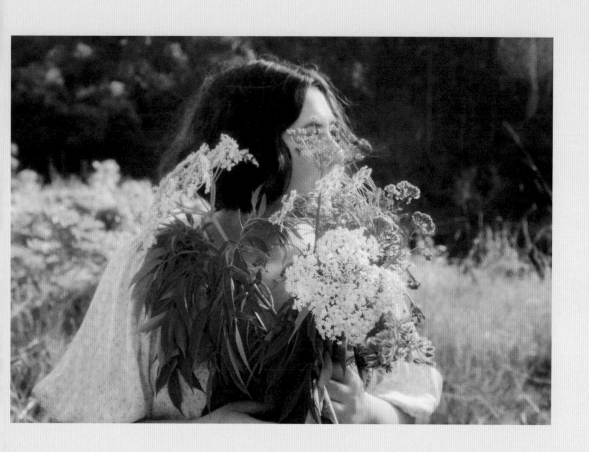

First published in Australia in 2020
by Thames & Hudson Australia Pty Ltd
11 Central Boulevard, Portside Business Park
Port Melbourne, Victoria 3207

ABN: 72 004 751 964

thamesandhudson.com.au

Text © Erin Lovell Verinder 2020
Images © Georgia Blackie 2020

23 22 21   5 4 3

The moral right of the author has been asserted.

All rights reserved. No part of this publication may be
reproduced or transmitted in any form or by any means,
electronic or mechanical, including photocopy, recording
or any other information storage or retrieval system,
without prior permission in writing from the publisher.

Any copy of this book issued by the publisher is sold
subject to the condition that it shall not by way of trade
or otherwise be lent, resold, hired out or otherwise
circulated without the publisher's prior consent in any
form or binding or cover other than that in which it is
published and without a similar condition including
these words being imposed on a subsequent purchaser.

Thames & Hudson Australia wishes to acknowledge that
Aboriginal and Torres Strait Islander people are the first
storytellers of this nation and the traditional custodians
of the land on which we live and work. We acknowledge
their continuing culture and pay respect to Elders past,
present and future.

978 1 760 76046 5 (hardback)
978 1 760 76169 1 (ebook)

 A catalogue record for this
book is available from the
National Library of Australia

Every effort has been made to trace accurate ownership
of copyrighted text and visual materials used in this
book. Errors or omissions will be corrected in subsequent
editions, provided notification is sent to the publisher.

Design: Alissa Dinallo
Editing: Sonja Heijn
Printed and bound in China by C&C Offset Printing Co., Ltd.

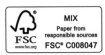

FSC® is dedicated to the promotion of responsible forest management
worldwide. This product is made of material from well-managed
FSC®-certified forests and other controlled sources.